Activity Schedules for Children with Autism

TOPICS IN AUTISM

SECOND EDITION

Activity Schedules for Children with Autism

TEACHING INDEPENDENT BEHAVIOR

**Lynn E. McClannahan, Ph.D.
& Patricia J. Krantz, Ph.D.**

Sandra L. Harris, Ph.D., series editor

Woodbine House ◆ 2010

© 1999, 2010 Lynn E. McClannahan and Patricia J. Krantz
Second edition

All rights reserved. Published in the United States of America by Woodbine House, Inc.,
6510 Bells Mill Road, Bethesda, MD 20817. 800-843-7323. www.woodbinehouse.com

Library of Congress Cataloging-in-Publication Data

McClannahan, Lynn E.
  Activity schedules for children with autism : teaching independent behavior / Lynn
E. McClannahan & Patricia J. Krantz. -- 2nd ed.
    p. cm.
  Includes bibliographical references and index.
  ISBN 978-1-60613-003-2
  1. Autistic children--Rehabilitation. 2. Autistic children--Education. 3. Autistic
children--Life skills guides. 4. Life skills--Study and teaching. I. Krantz, Patricia J.
II. Title.
  RJ506.A9M426 2010
  618.92'85882--dc22

                                                                      2010008842

Manufactured in the United States of America

10   9   8   7   6   5   4   3   2   1

This book is dedicated to
Professor Barbara Coleman Etzel
Teacher, researcher, and mentor

Table of Contents

Preface

Teaching youngsters with autism to use schedules is an exciting endeavor. We take pleasure in their steps toward independence, and admire their competence.

This book celebrates the accomplishments of many young people and their families. It is dedicated to the youngest children currently receiving intervention, who are learning picture-object correspondence skills. It is dedicated to children who, after becoming proficient schedule users, entered public school classrooms and put those skills to the test, managing homework assignments and changes in school routine. It is dedicated to children and adolescents who, although still receiving specialized intervention, contribute to family life by helping with household tasks, managing their own possessions, and initiating social interaction. And it is dedicated to adults with autism (some of them now in their 40s), whose proficient use of photographic or written activity schedules supports their independence in their homes and in community work places, where they make valued, and valuable, contributions.

We appreciate the participation of parents and professionals who, over the course of many years, have shared their experiences and their data about teaching young people to use activity schedules at home and in relatives' homes; at preschool or school; in places of worship; in dentists' and pediatricians' offices; in parks, playgrounds, and restaurants; and even during family vacations.

The intervention strategies described here are the product of a mutual endeavor with our friends and colleagues Gregory S. MacDuff and Edward C. Fenske. Our long-time cooperative relationships with them underlie the continued development of effective treatment systems that are supported by scientific data.

We thank the parents and professionals of IWRD (the Institute for Child Development), Gdansk, Poland, and TOHUM (the Foundation for Early Diagnosis and Education of Autism in Turkey) Istanbul, Turkey, for contributing photographs to this book. We celebrate their achievements.

1 | Independence, Choice, and Social Interaction

Tim

Chin in hand, Ellen watched her three-year-old son, Tim. Surrounded by new toys, he was lying on his back on the floor, rhythmically kicking a chair leg, humming, and staring at the ceiling light fixture. They had just finished a teaching session and he had performed well, pointing to pictures of familiar objects and imitating some sounds. But as soon as the session ended, he retreated to the floor. He looked neither at Ellen nor at the toys. Tired, she debated with herself about whether to prompt him to pick up a truck and roll it across the floor. He would probably object strenuously.

Jordan

As Jordan, age 7, happily finished his after-school snack, Dana braced herself for what was about to happen. She had promised her older son, Jack, that she would watch him ride his new bike—but she knew what Jordan would do when they approached the front door. Resolutely, she took him by the hand and said, as cheerfully as possible, "Let's go outside." As she opened the door, he screamed and fell on the threshold, kicking and crying. Jack, riding down the sidewalk, said, "I knew it!" As Dana struggled to move Jordan away from the door, she glimpsed Jack wheeling the bike into the garage.

Kris

Larry observed his adolescent daughter from a vantage point slightly obscured by the kitchen door. Kris was still sitting on the couch, doing absolutely nothing. He continued to watch her inactivity as he reflected. She attended a good education program, and she had learned a lot. She knew how to make her bed, bathe, fold laundry, make her own school lunch, and play a variety of computer games, and she usually did her homework without much assistance. But she would do none of these unless he stood up, walked toward her, and gave a direction, such as, "Why don't you fix your lunch for tomorrow?"

Introduction

Tim, Jordan, and Kris strike a familiar chord for many of us. Tim, a preschooler, displays his new skills in structured teaching sessions, but has not learned how to appropriately fill the less-structured times between activities. Jordan is often pleasant and endearing when following familiar family routines, but tantrums occur when his routines are changed. And Kris, who has acquired many competencies, does nothing unless instructed by her parents or teachers. Carefully planned activity schedules can help solve these problems and many others.

Background

This book is based on more than two decades of research conducted at the Princeton Child Development Institute. In 1986, we began our studies because we observed that, although children and youths with autism were learning many things, they frequently failed to display their skills unless someone gave a verbal instruction, modeled the desired behavior, or gestured toward materials. Sometimes, even the smallest prompts (a half-step toward a child, or an expectant look) enabled them to do the activities. But when prompts from adults were absent, they displayed stereotypy; that is, they engaged in finger play, hand flapping, vocal noise, twirling round and round, noncontextual laughter, or other repetitive behavior, or they simply waited.

We did not assume that the children were "wrong" or incapable of using the skills they had learned—instead, we assumed that it was important to examine different teaching procedures to enable them to perform activities and tasks independently.

What Is an Activity Schedule?

An activity schedule is a set of pictures or words that cues someone to engage in a sequence of activities. An activity schedule can take many forms, but initially it is usually a three-ring binder with pictures or words on each page that cue children to perform tasks, engage in activities, or enjoy rewards. Depending on the child, the activity can be very detailed—breaking a task into all of its separate parts—or it can be very general, using one picture or symbol to cue a child to perform an entire task or activity. Through graduated guidance (discussed below), children are taught to open their schedule books, turn to the first page, perform the task, and then turn to the next page for cues to the next task. The goal of teaching schedule use is to enable children with autism to perform tasks and activities without direct prompting and guidance by parents or teachers.

The schedule book for Riley, age 2, contains five pages, each of which displays one picture. The pictures show a frame-tray puzzle, a color-matching game, balls that fit in a plastic tube, felt animal cut-outs and a felt board, and corn chips on a paper plate. When his mother or instructor says "It's time to play with toys," Riley opens his picture book, points to the first picture, goes to a nearby bookcase and gets a basket that contains the puzzle shown on page one, brings the puzzle to his little table, puts the pieces in their respective places, returns the puzzle to the basket, puts the basket back on the shelf, returns to his picture book, turns the page, points to the color-matching task, and so on. The teaching procedures enable Riley to do five activities without help from his parents or instructors. Although still a toddler, he engages in independent play for ten to fifteen minutes. Before he learned to use his picture schedule, he did not play—instead, he briefly picked up toys and mouthed them, then dropped them and went on to do the same with other play materials.

Page, age 12, read at the second-grade level, and quickly acquired new sight words. After school, she followed a written schedule—a list

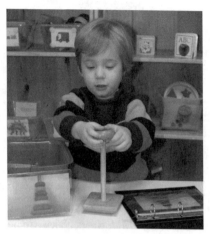

(Fig. 1-1) At 26 months, Sean is learning to complete his first photographic activity schedule, which contains five pictures. Note that his schedule book is nearby, and is open to the page that displays the picture of the stacking rings.

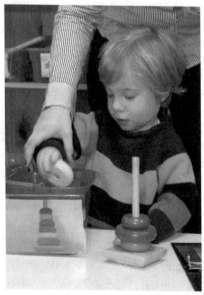

(Fig. 1-2) Because he has not yet mastered this task, his teacher steps forward to use a prompting procedure called graduated guidance. (This procedure is discussed in Chapter 4.)

of activities to be accomplished. Some of the activities on her list were: vacuum my room, reading homework, make pudding, fold towels, math homework, piano, exercise video, set table. Page pointed to the first item on the list ("vacuum my room"), obtained the necessary materials, and began. After completing each activity, she returned to her schedule and placed a check mark beside that item. Before new activities were added to Page's schedule, her teachers presented the new words on flash cards, and helped her learn to read them.

Many of the activities in Page's schedule were originally taught as separate lists; for example, in an earlier version of her activity schedule, the task of making pudding was separated into nineteen written instructions, such as "get milk," "get bowl," and "get pudding mix." Following a written activity schedule enabled Page to use after-school time to practice new skills and to help with household tasks. Before she became a proficient schedule follower, she often spent after-school hours making perseverative demands on family members, and screaming if she did not get her way.

Independence

Riley and Page are examples of the independence that children gain when they learn to follow activity schedules. Riley's mother no longer has to monitor him continuously and remove toys from his mouth, and Page's parents don't have to give constant verbal instruction or respond to her repetitive demands. The activity schedules decreased the need for adult prompting and guidance. These results were achieved with special teaching procedures.

One of our first investigations of activity schedules (MacDuff, Krantz, & McClannahan, 1993) was conducted in one of the Princeton Child Development Institute's family-style group homes. The four boys (ages 9 to 14) who participated in the study had learned many home-living skills, such as vacuuming, dusting, table setting, doing puzzles, playing with toys, and riding bikes. But they did not do these activities unless verbally instructed, and when staff members' prompts were withdrawn, the boys were often "off-task"—not engaged in any appropriate activity.

Using a teaching procedure called graduated guidance, we taught the boys to follow photographic activity schedules that depicted six different leisure and homework activities, such as Lego blocks, Perfection game, handwriting worksheets, and Tinker Toys. For example, when a youth turned to a page of his schedule book that displayed a picture of a Tinker Toy car, he learned to point to the picture, take the Tinker Toys off the shelf above his desk, assemble the car as shown in the picture, put the Tinker Toys back in the box, return the box to the shelf, and turn to the next picture in his schedule. Because these boys already knew all the steps necessary to complete each activity, their activity schedules did not cue them to do each separate step, although for other children we often create activity schedules that do that.

When the boys were doing the activities depicted in their schedule books without much help, we carefully faded the instructor's guidance, and, finally, his presence. Near the end of the study, although we changed the order of the photographs and even added new photographs, the boys continued to follow their schedules without prompts from adults and, on average, they were "on-task" or appropriately engaged during 91% to 99% of our observations.

These boys, who previously experienced considerable difficulty in pursuing and finishing activities, and in making transitions from one activity to the next, now independently completed six different activities without adult help! They looked very competent.

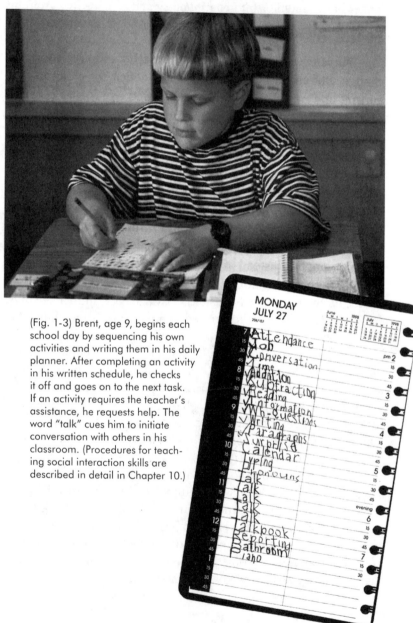

(Fig. 1-3) Brent, age 9, begins each school day by sequencing his own activities and writing them in his daily planner. After completing an activity in his written schedule, he checks it off and goes on to the next task. If an activity requires the teacher's assistance, he requests help. The word "talk" cues him to initiate conversation with others in his classroom. (Procedures for teaching social interaction skills are described in detail in Chapter 10.)

Choice

Imagine yourself transported to another culture. You do not understand the language spoken there, and do not have a guide or translator. People ask you where you would like to go and what you would like to do, but you cannot comprehend or respond to these questions. This scenario describes the plight of many youngsters with autism who, because of their severe language deficits, are unable to participate in decisions about their own activities and daily schedules. Not surprisingly, this lack of control over the events of daily life often appears to be associated with tantrums and disruptive behavior—we would probably tantrum too if we were never allowed to decide when to eat, what task to do next, or which leisure activity to select.

Photographic and written activity schedules provide a framework for helping children with autism learn to make choices. If we provide careful and systematic instruction, they not only learn to follow schedules, but they also learn to sequence their own activities, and to choose leisure activities that follow structured teaching sessions, homework, or home-living tasks.

Social Interaction

Pursuing our daily activities inevitably requires social exchange. But social interaction is a key deficit for children with autism, and one that should be addressed as soon as possible. Although discrete-trial training is often used to teach children with autism to imitate words, phrases, and sentences and to make verbal responses when requested to do so, this approach is not representative of the give-and-take of ordinary conversation. In discrete-trial teaching, the parent or teacher asks a question or gives an instruction and waits for the child to respond. And youngsters learn to respond and then wait for the next instruction. Indeed, many children appear to become dependent upon adults' verbal prompts—instead of initiating social interaction, they wait for others to do so. But in typical conversation, either partner may initiate, often with observations or comments, rather than with questions or directions, and one person may make several statements before the other replies.

Teaching children to use activity schedules creates a different framework for building social interaction skills, and sets many occasions for children to initiate conversation, rather than merely responding to others' instructions or queries. We recommend that even the first schedule for the youngest preschooler include at least one simple interaction task. A child who has not yet acquired language may learn to point to a picture in a schedule book and approach a parent for a toss in the air; a youngster who now has a few words may seek out a family member to say "Hi" or request "Tickle"; and a boy or girl who uses sentences may initiate conversation by requesting a preferred activity ("I want hug"), or reporting on a recently completed activity ("I did puzzle").

Our experience in early intervention programs, preschool, school, and group homes indicates that social interaction activities should be included in every activity schedule, and should be extended and elaborated as soon as possible. This theme will reappear in several subsequent chapters, together with specific suggestions about how to use activity schedules to build conversation skills.

We All Use Schedules

We are busy people. We have many commitments and we use schedules to help us accomplish our various responsibilities. We use appointment books, day timers, planners, or calendars. We use "to-do" lists that we post on the refrigerator or keep in a pocket, wallet, or purse. Some of us use electronic appointment books or computer software to keep track of our obligations.

Photographic and written activity schedules serve precisely the same function for children, youths, and adults with autism. Schedules remind them of the tasks that must be accomplished so that they, like us, need not depend upon other persons to instruct or "nag" about things that need to be done.

We would be very reluctant to give up our appointment books. Similarly, we do not ask young people with autism to give up their schedules. Instead, we help them acquire skills that enable them to use schedules that are increasingly like our own. Later we will discuss teaching procedures that help children make the transition from photographic to written schedules and from written schedules to day timers, appointment books, or pocket computers.

About This Book

This book is designed to introduce you to activity schedules and guide you as a parent or professional as you teach your child with autism to follow an activity schedule. Although many of the examples pertain to children, we have also included examples relevant to adolescents and adults. It is never too late to help your son or daughter or student become more independent.

Chapter 2 discusses the skills that young people need before they begin first activity schedules, and explains how to teach these important prerequisites. Chapter 3 describes how to construct an activity schedule that is especially suited to your child's strengths. Chapter 4 provides detailed information about the teaching procedures, and Chapter 5 shows you how to measure your child's schedule-following skills. Chapter 6 explains what to do after your child masters the first schedule (with special emphasis on changing the sequence of photographs, adding new photographs, and gradually decreasing supervision). Chapter 7 addresses activities that have no clear ending (watching TV, for example), and describes how to help your child learn when to end one activity and move on to the next. Chapter 8 explains how to teach children to select their own rewards and sequence their own activities, and Chapter 9 takes a look at how children learn to follow written, rather than pictorial schedules. Chapter 10 focuses on using activity schedules to expand social interaction skills, Chapter 11 discusses how activity schedules are helpful to adults with autism, and Chapter 12 explains how activity schedules provide an organizational framework that expands young people's independence, competence, and choice. Finally, Chapter 13 suggests solutions to the problems that sometimes arise when we teach children, youths, and adults to use activity schedules.

Time and effort are required to construct children's schedules, to teach them to follow schedules, and to systematically decrease supervision, so that they can learn to be more independent and productive and spend less time engaging in dysfunctional behavior (Krantz, MacDuff, & McClannahan, 1993). Many parents and teachers are already investing a great deal of time and effort in providing continuous supervision, correcting children who are off-task, and responding to disruptive behavior. Making a comparable investment in teaching photographic or written activity schedules gives young people key skills that are of lifelong importance.

Gordie

After returning the coloring book and crayons to a bookcase, Gordie turned a page of his schedule book and studied the next photograph, a picture of him and his sister eating cookies. His sister Gwen, age 8, glanced in his direction and interrupted the game she was playing with a friend to confide, "My brother used to ignore me, but now he talks to me, sometimes." Entering the kitchen, Gordie said, "Mom, cookies please." Seconds later, with cookies in hand, he approached his sister and said, "Cookies!"

Elliott

Elliott waved goodbye to his job coach, entered his apartment, went directly to his desk, and opened his appointment book to a paper-clipped page. The first item on his written schedule that he had not yet checked off was "take out trash." Returning from the dumpster a few minutes later, he put a check mark by that item and read the next, "iron work shirts and pants." Before going to get the ironing board, he glanced down the list and read, "call grandpa" and "plan menus."

2 | Prerequisite Skills: Is My Child Ready for an Activity Schedule?

Introduction

Children must learn certain skills, such as distinguishing a picture of an object from a background and matching identical objects, before they can learn to use activity schedules. Other skills not critical to learning to use activity schedules, such as putting materials away, can be acquired at the same time a child is learning to follow a schedule. This chapter discusses the skills that are necessary and makes suggestions about how to teach them; it also describes other skills that are likely to facilitate teaching and learning.

Identifying Picture versus Background

Some youngsters with autism may not yet have learned that, when presented with a picture or photograph mounted on a plain background, they should attend to the picture and not the background. Of course, in order to follow photographic activity schedules, children must learn that it is the pictures, not the backgrounds, that require scrutiny. You can assess your child's skills in this area by making a simple book, using construction paper and self-adhesive stickers that depict familiar objects. Put ten pieces of construction paper (all the same color) in a three-ring binder. Then apply one sticker per page—but put each sticker in a different location. For example, the sticker on page one may be in the upper-left corner, the sticker on page two may be in the middle of the page, and so on. Slide each page into a plastic page protector. These are useful because they extend the life of the book, and they also discourage children from attempting to remove the stickers.

Sit beside your child at a table or desk, open the book to page one, and ask, "Where's the picture?" or say, "Point to the picture." Wait five seconds, and then mark "plus" (+) on a data sheet (see Figure 2-1 and Appendix A) if your child touched the sticker during that time, or "minus" (–) if he did not touch the sticker. Score the first response your child makes on each page; for example, if he touches the background first, and then touches the sticker, score minus. If your youngster touches the stickers on at least eight of the ten pages, you can probably assume that picture-versus-background skills have already been acquired.

If your son or daughter cannot yet do this task, you can teach it. Reserve a special snack or toy for those times when you will look at the sticker book together, and plan to do this activity several times each

Fig. 2-1 | Identifying Picture versus Background Data Sheet for Duane

Opportunity #	Task	Date/Time	Date/Time	Date/Time
	Picture versus Background	1/18/10 11 a.m.	1/18/10 4 p.m.	1/19/10 4:30 p.m.
1		–	–	+
2		–	–	–
3		+	–	+
4		+	+	+
5		–	–	+
6		–	+	–
7		–	+	+
8		–	+	+
9		+	+	+
10		+	+	+
Number Correct		4	6	8

(Fig. 2–1) Sample data sheet used to measure a child's skills in identifying picture versus background. Blank data sheets are included in Appendix A.

day. After you say, "Point to the picture," try to anticipate your child's response, so that you can prevent errors by gently but quickly guiding his hand to the sticker. If you have to help, give lots of enthusiastic praise ("Good, you found the picture"), but don't provide the preferred toy or snack—reserve these for the occasions when he makes a correct response all by himself.

Throughout this book, there are many references to edible rewards, such as raisins, popcorn, and cereal. Early in intervention, many youngsters with autism do not value praise, attention, or toys, and preferred snacks may therefore be important rewards. However, if your child enjoys stickers, stars, coins, or activities such as patty cake, peek-a-boo, or tickles, it is certainly appropriate to use these as rewards.

Matching Identical Objects

Children who are fluent and successful schedule-followers have learned that a picture of an object corresponds to an object. For example, a picture of a Big Bird toy represents the stuffed toy. But before they learn picture-object correspondence skills, children learn matching skills; that is, they learn to identify objects that are identical. It is often easier for youngsters with autism to learn to match identical three-dimensional objects, such as two bananas or two cups, before they learn to match two-dimensional objects, such as two identical stickers, or two cut-out red circles.

To determine whether your child can match identical objects, sit with her at a table or desk, and arrange five different toys or household objects on the work surface. Put five identical objects out of her sight (in your lap or pocket, or on the floor beside you). Display one of your objects (for example, a spoon) on the tabletop and say, "Point." After she points to the object you placed directly in front of her say, "Find." If your youngster reaches for, touches, or picks up the matching object within five seconds of your instruction, score this as a correct response (see Figure 2-2 on the next page and Appendix A). If she does not respond, responds after five seconds, or touches the wrong object before touching or picking up the correct object, score an incorrect response. Continue until you have provided ten opportunities for matching. Children who have learned matching skills can usually make correct responses on eight of ten opportunities; some errors may occur because

Fig. 2-2 | Matching Identical Objects
Data Sheet for Judy

Opportunity #	Task	Date/Time	Date/Time	Date/Time
	Matching Identical Objects	1/27/10 3:45 p.m.	1/28/10 4:00 p.m.	1/29/10 4:30 p.m.
1	Sock	−	−	−
2	Spoon	−	+	+
3	Ball	+	+	+
4	Pencil	+	+	+
5	Bar of soap	−	−	−
6	Ball	+	+	+
7	Sock	−	+	+
8	Pencil	+	+	+
9	Bar of soap	−	−	−
10	Spoon	+	−	+
Number Correct		5	6	7

(Fig. 2–2) Sample data sheet used to measure a child's skills in matching identical objects. Blank data sheets are included in Appendix A.

of inattention. If your child hasn't yet learned to match identical objects, you can teach her by using the manual guidance, praise, and special rewards procedures described above.

Picture-Object Correspondence Skills

A child who has picture-object correspondence skills has learned that pictures represent depicted objects. These skills are central to the use of photographic activity schedules, but many children with autism require special instruction to help them learn the relationships between objects and pictures.

In order to measure your child's skills, make another "book" by placing five pieces of construction paper (all the same color) in a three-ring binder. Then photograph five familiar objects or cut out five magazine pictures, mount one on each page of the book, and collect five objects that are identical to those in the pictures. For example, you may find a picture of your child's favorite beverage, and purchase a bottle of that beverage. A toy catalog may contain a picture of a doll or car that is among your child's toys. Or an advertising circular may show a picture of a towel that is identical to your towels. The objects you collect should be exactly the same as those in the pictures, and each picture should show only the target object, and no other objects.

Sit beside your child and put the book and the objects on a work surface in front of him. Open the book, and model by pointing to the first picture, while you say, "Point." If necessary, guide your child's hand to help him point to the picture. Then say, "Find," and guide your child to pick up the target object. Immediately after he picks up an object that corresponds to the picture, praise him and give him special attention—for example, clap for him, whistle, toss him in the air, or give him a hug, kiss, or tickle. Repeat this procedure on each page of the book.

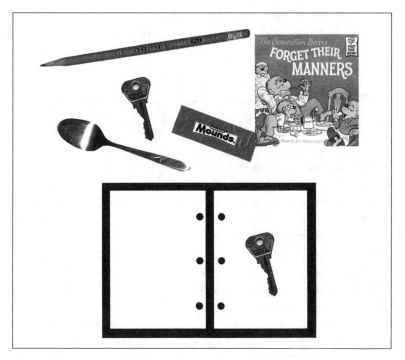

(Fig. 2-3) To teach picture-object correspondence, model pointing to the picture, say "Point," and guide the child's hand to point to the picture. Then say "Find," and guide the child to pick up the corresponding object and place it on the page.

The next time you use the book, give the instructions "Point" and "Find," and wait five seconds for your child to respond. Score his responses correct if he points and finds the target object within five seconds and without your help; score incorrect if he does not point within five seconds, does not pick up the target object, or picks up an object that does not correspond to the picture (see Figure 2-4 and Appendix A).

Fig. 2-4	Picture-Object Correspondence Data Sheet for Roger				
Opportunity #	**Task**	**Date/Time**	**Date/Time**	**Date/Time**
	Picture–Object Correspondence	2/9/10 5 p.m.	2/9/10 7 p.m.	2/10/10 4:30 p.m.
1	Truck	−	−	−
2	Cup	−	+	+
3	Shoe	−	−	−
4	Block	−	−	+
5	Toothbrush	+	+	+
Number Correct		1	2	3

(Fig. 2–4) Sample data sheet used to measure a child's picture–object correspondence skills. Blank data sheets are included in Appendix A.

If your youngster does not make correct responses on at least three of the five tasks, you will probably want to use the book to teach picture-object correspondence. Return to the procedures you used when you first introduced the book. Model pointing to the picture and guide your child to point to it and then pick up the corresponding object; follow this with enthusiastic praise and attention. Over a period of time, gradually withdraw your guidance. When he finds an object without your help, give him a special snack or toy, as well as praise and affection.

When your child makes correct responses on each page, it is time for a new book. Select different pictures and objects, and measure your son's responses the first time you present the new book. If he does not respond correctly on three of the five pages, continue to teach until he can do all of the tasks in the second book without your help. Continue to make new books and assess his progress until he achieves at least three of five correct responses the first time you present a new book.

Accepting Manual Guidance

The procedures we use to teach children to follow activity schedules emphasize manual guidance. If we are to accomplish this teaching, children must permit us to touch their hands, arms, and shoulders, and must allow us to guide them. Many youngsters do not display any signs of discomfort when they are physically guided by a parent or teacher, but a few respond by screaming, crying, resisting, or attempting to flee.

Observe your child when you are assisting her with tasks she has not yet mastered, such as putting her shoes on, pulling up her underwear, brushing her teeth, or using a spoon. Does she object if you put your hands over hers and help her with these activities? Children who appear comfortable with this type of assistance usually respond well to the type of instruction used in teaching activity schedules.

If your child resists manual guidance, there are several things you can do to teach her to be more receptive to your help. What kind of physical contact does she enjoy? If she likes tickles, piggyback rides, tosses in the air, or being rocked in your lap, try to introduce a small amount of manual guidance each time you share these activities, and gradually increase your guidance over a period of days. For example, take her hand and show her how to tickle you before you tickle her. Or manually guide her to climb on a bed or chair before you begin the piggyback ride.

You may also want to pair your manual guidance with preferred toys or snacks. Guide her hand to pick up a special snack food, and gradually increase your physical contact over time. Put a special toy on a high shelf, and, as you lift her up, guide her hand to reach for it. On each of these occasions, try to use the maximum amount of manual guidance that your child can tolerate without exhibiting unwanted behavior such as resisting, crying, or hitting. These tactics ultimately enable most children to accept manual prompts. When you teach new skills such as those described in this and subsequent chapters, remember to use manual guidance not only when preventing or correcting errors, but also when delivering rewards and engaging in your child's preferred activities.

Using Materials

It is helpful if a preschooler can string beads or complete puzzles, but these skills are not essential to the introduction of first photographic activity schedules. In fact, youngsters often acquire new work or play skills at the same time that they learn to follow activity schedules. But your child may learn more quickly if you can identify some activities that he has already mastered. Can he put shapes in a shape box? Can he sort picture cards into categories? Can he put knives, forks, and spoons in their respective places in the kitchen drawer? If he can do these or similar tasks, you may want to include them in his first schedule. Steven, age 3, had learned to drop blocks in a toy mailbox, to sort plastic horses and sheep into separate containers, and to assemble nesting cups. By including these familiar tasks in his first photographic activity schedule, his teacher made it easier for him to develop schedule-following skills.

Summary

In this chapter, we made some suggestions about how to measure and if necessary teach prerequisite skills that help a child begin a first photographic activity schedule. But there are many ways to begin. We know some young people who simultaneously learned picture-object correspondence skills and schedule-following skills. Although it took them longer to master their first schedules, they are competent schedule users today. However, time spent teaching children to identify picture versus background, to match identical objects, and to identify objects that correspond to pictures is typically time well-invested, because these skills facilitate schedule following.

3 | Preparing a First Activity Schedule

Brook

Before her teacher constructed her first schedule, Brook, age 6, had already learned to put pegs in the Lite Brite, to color simple shapes, and to give someone a "high five," but she only engaged in these activities when instructed by someone to do so. Her first schedule book included five photographs. The first three pictures showed: 1) the Lite Brite and pegs, 2) crayons and a page to be colored, and 3) Brook giving a teacher a "high five." Two other photographs showed unfamiliar activities: 4) bristle blocks and 5) raisins on a paper plate. The photographs were mounted in her schedule book, one picture to a page, and the actual materials depicted in the photos were arranged on a bookshelf near her desk.

After a few weeks of teaching, Brook dependably responded to her teacher's instruction to "Find something to do"; she opened her schedule book, pointed to the first picture, got the Lite Brite and pegs from a container on the bookshelf, assembled the pegs to create a picture, put the materials away, returned to her schedule, turned the page, pointed to the picture of crayons, and so on. After pointing to the picture of "high five," she approached her teacher with hand raised, and her teacher used this interaction to provide praise and attention. When she arrived at the last photograph in the book, Brook brought the paper plate to her desk, ate the raisins, and threw the paper plate in the wastebasket. Previously she was unable to do any activities without teachers' assistance; using her first photographic activity schedule, she remained appropriately engaged with play and learning activities for about twenty minutes.

Selecting Activities

Children learn schedule-following skills more rapidly if some of the activities in the first schedule are familiar or already mastered. It is also helpful to keep the initial schedule brief; plan to begin with no more than four or five activities.

A first photographic schedule for a preschooler might include a frame-tray puzzle, stacking cups, requesting a toss in the air, shapes and shape box, and a preferred snack. A schedule for a six- or seven-year-old might include work and play activities such as tracing lines on a worksheet; arranging letters or numerals in sequence on a magnetic board; requesting a tickle; assembling a toy such as a Lego car or a Mr. Potato Head; and having a preferred snack. And a first schedule for a ten-year-old might include some typical after-school activities, such as hanging up his jacket; using the toilet; washing his hands; putting away items in his lunchbox (for example, putting the thermos on the kitchen counter, food containers in the dishwasher, and cold pack in the freezer); reporting that he has put things away; and getting his own after-school snack. It is important to select activities that are age-appropriate, so that when your child or student is independently following his schedule, he will appear skillful and competent.

You should also select activities that have clear endings, so that your youngster will know when each task is completed. A frame-tray puzzle is completed when all of the pieces are in place; a pegboard activity is finished when all the pegs are in the board (you can adjust the difficulty of this task by supplying a larger or smaller number of pegs). A worksheet is finished when all the trac-

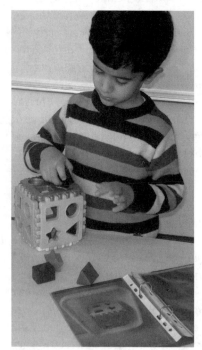

(Fig. 3-1) In Istanbul, Osman, age 5, follows a photographic schedule without help.

ing tasks are done, or when all of the shapes are colored, and you can adjust task length and complexity when you construct the worksheet.

In selecting activities, you may rely on local toy stores or school supply catalogs, or you may create curriculum materials that are relevant to your family, or that reflect your child's current skills and interests. For example, using tag board or file folders and Velcro, you can design matching tasks (mounting the letters "M, "o," and "m" over identical letters that are displayed under a photograph of mother). Or, you can design numeral-object correspondence tasks (mounting the numeral "2" by a picture of two dogs, and the numeral "5" by a picture of five dinosaurs).

The first schedule should end with a snack or play activity that is especially enjoyable for your child. It is best to reserve this special treat for those times when your child is using his schedule; do not make this preferred food or activity available at other times.

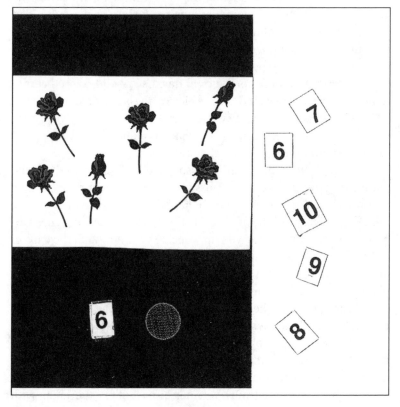

(Fig. 3-2) A numeral-object correspondence task.

After you have identified the activities that will be included in the first schedule, consider how to make it easy for your youngster to pick them up and put them away. Plastic dishpans, plastic baskets, or shoeboxes are often helpful in packaging materials so that young children are less likely to drop them. These containers minimize the loss of small pieces, and assist children in learning to return materials to designated locations.

Taking Pictures

You don't have to be a photographer to take the pictures that will be displayed in the schedule, but a few simple rules are important. Photographs should show only the target materials or activity, and should not include objects or events that might be confusing or distracting. Materials should be photographed against a plain background, and target objects should almost fill the frame. And pictures that are over- or under-exposed or out of focus should be discarded.

If you aren't an experienced photographer, you may find it helpful to take pictures outdoors on a bright day. Use a solid-colored carpet remnant, a piece of plywood, a large piece of tag board or foam board, a solid-colored table top, a sidewalk, or some other nonreflective surface to create a plain background. Light shade is helpful in getting a good exposure without getting your shadow in the picture.

Arrange all of the materials associated with one activity on the plain background and, when possible, arrange them to show how they are used. For example, you might photograph a five-piece puzzle with four pieces, and the fifth beside the puzzle. If stacking cups will be kept in a plastic basket, you may decide to photograph the cups in or beside the basket, or you may show some of the cups in the basket and others beside it. If a preschooler's snack is a few M&M's on a paper plate, photograph the candy on the plate, just as it will be presented. If a ten-year-old will get her own snack, photograph the full juice glass, the cookies, and the cookie plate that you want her to obtain.

Professional photographers "bracket" their exposures—that is, they take one picture at what appears to be the best camera setting, and then take two more at faster or slower shutter speeds, or larger or smaller lens aperture settings. You may also want to experiment with several shots of the same materials, and later select the best picture.

Digital cameras and printers make it easy to store and re-use photographs, and many parents and professionals maintain libraries of photographs. Commercially available photo libraries (e.g., Silver Lining Multimedia, 2000; Stages Learning Materials, 1997) are also helpful. Although a child masters her first schedule and goes on to new activities and materials, components of previous schedules may later be used to construct special schedules that can be used during vacation travel, visits to the pediatrician's office, or trips to relatives' homes. A photograph of a Lego car to be assembled may be removed from a youngster's schedule book and replaced with a photograph of a more complex model-building task, but the old picture and materials may become part of a schedule that is used at Grandma's house.

Preparing Materials

After you have collected the materials for the activity schedule, assemble them. Depending upon your child's size, age, and motor skills, you may decide to display the photographs in a 9-by-12 or a 7-by-9-inch binder, or even in a small photo album. Three-ring binders are useful because they lay flat when open, so that a child does not "lose his place."

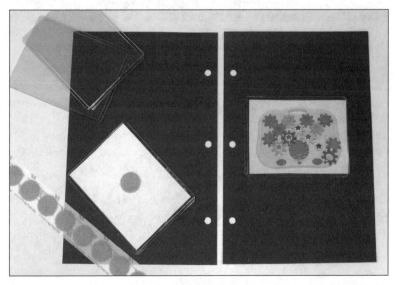

(Fig. 3-3) A first photographic activity schedule. The pictures are encased in plastic baseball card holders, and the holders are attached to schedule pages with Velcro.

Insert pieces of construction paper into four or five plastic page protectors, and put the page protectors in the binder. All pages should be identical, so that the color of the page, or other irrelevant stimuli will not interfere with your child's attention to the pictures. Place each picture in a plastic sleeve; clear plastic baseball card holders, available from hobby shops, are convenient for this purpose.

Finally, attach a Velcro circle or square to the center of each binder page, attach the matching Velcro to the back of each plastic photo holder, and mount the pictures in the schedule book. This will make it possible to change the order of the photographs after your child has mastered a first schedule. We discuss the importance of resequencing photographs in Chapter 6.

Select an activity sequence that offers variety. Children's interest may flag if they are asked to do three puzzles, or complete four pages of connecting the dots. If a child will do two worksheet tasks, separate them with a different activity, such as folding towels or building a model. And remember, the preferred snack or activity should be the last picture in the schedule.

Fig. 3-4 | Preparing a First Activity Schedule
Materials Needed

Schedule
- Camera and film or digital camera and printer
- Nonreflective background
- Materials to be included in the schedule
- Three-ring binder or album
- Plastic page protectors
- Construction paper
- Velcro circles or squares
- Photographs
- Baseball card holders

Token System
- Clipboard
- Coins, stars, stickers, or happy faces
- Velcro circles

Social Interaction Activities
- Button-activated voice recorders*
- Card reader and cards*

Home Environment
- Bookcases, shelves, or desk surface
- Bins, baskets, dishpans, or shoeboxes

---

*Button-activated voice recorders (see Appendix B) and card readers (see Appendix C) are optional; it is possible to substitute photographs or text.

Identifying and Preparing Rewards

What rewards does your youngster presently enjoy? Does she receive bites of favorite foods as rewards for good performance? Is she accustomed to stars, stickers, happy faces, or other types of token rewards? You can begin a first activity schedule even if your child has not yet learned to value tokens, but her progress will be more rapid if you teach her to use a token system.

There are many advantages associated with the use of coins as tokens. This reinforcement procedure teaches children to value money, and can also be used to teach them to identify and count coins, and to use an allowance system like the one you may use with your other children. (Of course, if your youngster puts small objects in her mouth, you should select larger tokens, such as poker chips, blocks, or puzzle pieces).

Teaching a child to use a token system can often be accomplished in only a few sessions. Select a familiar teaching activity, and use rewards that you typically deliver. Perhaps you are teaching your child to point to or label pictures of family members, pictures of common objects, or alphabet letters, and you reward correct responses with musical toys and bites of cookie or pretzel. Conduct your teaching session as usual, but when your child makes a correct response, give her a coin and quickly say, "Give me a penny, and I'll give you cookie," while manually guiding this exchange. As soon as possible, ask for two responses and give your daughter a penny after each response before making the exchange. Then gradually increase the number of pennies needed to obtain the cookie, pretzel, or toy.

Your child will learn to value coins as a result of the consistent pairing of a preferred item (bites of cookie) and a new item (pennies). By gradually in-

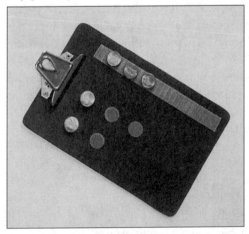

(Fig. 3-5) A token system that uses pennies. Pennies are attached to the clipboard with Velcro.

creasing the number of pennies needed for an exchange, you will help to counteract performance problems that occur when a child tires of the available rewards. There are limits on the number of cookies or pretzels any of us wants to consume on a given occasion.

To construct a monetary token system, purchase a small (6-inch by 9-inch) clipboard and find the pennies that accumulate in your purse or dresser drawer. Attach circular adhesive Velcro hooks to the back of each penny, and place the adhesive Velcro loops on the clipboard. Use the number of pennies that your child typically earns before exchanging tokens for a preferred food, toy, or activity. Placing a strip of Velcro on the edge of the clipboard provides a convenient way to store the pennies when they are not in use.

Alternatively, you might use plastic letters or numbers as tokens. Some children learn to identify alphabet letters or count if the teacher says, "A!" or "You earned B" when delivering alphabet letters or says, "Number one!" or "Two!" when delivering plastic numerals. When used as tokens, laminated photographs of family members, animals, or favorite cartoon characters may not only enhance a child's interest, but also teach additional language skills.

Designing the Environment

A goal for many parents is teaching children to pick up after themselves, and to put things away. This is a reasonable expectation for your son with autism, as well as for his siblings. But children cannot put things away if they do not know where toys, clothing, food, and learning materials belong. Teaching your child to follow a first activity schedule presents an opportunity to teach him that the materials he uses should be returned to designated places. Helping him acquire this important skill requires organizing his living and learning environment.

Before you begin to teach schedule following, identify an appropriate setting (his classroom, his bedroom, the living room, or the family room) and make materials easily accessible by placing them (in sequence, from left to right) on a shelf, bookcase, table, or desk. Materials should be within the child's reach, and there should be ample space to return a basket or box to the shelf after completing an activity. If space is not currently available, you may want to purchase a bookcase or some shelving. If you plan to teach an after-school schedule (described above), identify kitchen cupboards, drawers, and refrigerator shelves where plates, cookies, napkins, and juice will always reside.

Preparing to Teach Social Interaction Skills

Gordon, a preschooler with autism, offers some examples of how to include social interaction in activity schedules. At two years of age, he learned to follow his first photographic activity schedule. A picture of blowing bubbles was mounted in his schedule book, and because he had not yet learned to talk, he was taught to remove the photograph from his book and present it to his mother or father, who responded with simple language models ("Bubbles!" or "Bubbles are fun!") and then blew bubbles that Gordon enjoyed catching.

By the time he was three, Gordon had learned to imitate words and phrases and his instructors began to use miniature button-activated voice recorders when they added social activities to his schedule. They pre-recorded words, using a pen to depress the record

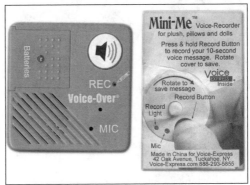

(Fig. 3-6) Button-activated voice recorders. See Appendix B for ordering information.

button while saying those words. Photographs that cued social activities were attached to pages of Gordon's schedule book. One page displayed a photograph of a favorite toy, a tiger hand puppet. Gordon learned to point to the picture, find the nearby puppet and an attached voice recorder, and press the button on the recorder, which played the previously recorded word "Look." When he approached a teacher with the puppet and imitated the recording, his teachers responded with language that he could understand, such as "Tigers say 'rrr'!" Then they provided rewards—tickles, bounces, and tosses in the air.

Chapter 1 discussed the importance of including social interaction tasks in activity schedules. There are several ways to accomplish this. Social exchanges, like other activities, can be represented by photo-

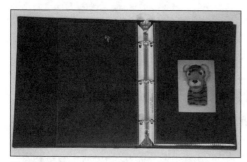

(Fig. 3-7a) Gordon's schedule contains a picture of a puppet.

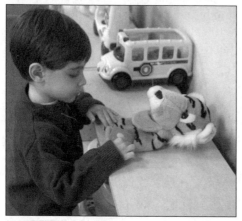

(Fig. 3-7b) He finds the puppet and an attached button-activated recorder and presses the button to play the script "Look."

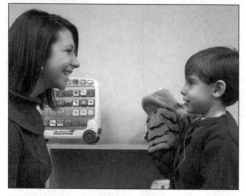

(Fig. 3-7c) Then he takes the puppet to his nearby instructor and says, "Look."

graphs. For example, a picture of a child with one hand raised may cue a greeting, such as waving "Hi"; a picture of a child standing in front of a parent and raising both hands may signal a toss in the air; and a picture of a piggy-back ride may indicate that it is time for the youngster to approach a family member for a ride. With these pictures, children who have not yet acquired speech can initiate and participate in social activities.

If your youngster has learned to read some sight words, you may use text to cue social interaction. Words such as "juice" or "tickle" might indicate that the child should approach you and say, "I want juice" or "Tickle, please." Or if reading skills have progressed sufficiently, the schedule may include short sentences, such as "I'm done," "I finished my worksheets," or "Look at my picture."

In our experience, many children who are learning to follow first activity schedules have not yet learned to read, and are just beginning to talk. Although they may imitate a few words, they do not engage in spontaneous speech or initiate social interaction, and these are important goals. For these children, button-activated voice recorders or card readers are often components of activity schedules.

The card reader is a tape recorder and player that operates with special cards upon which a strip of

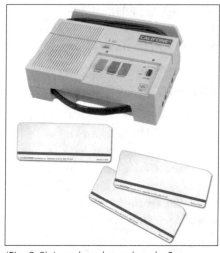

(Fig. 3-8) A card reader and cards. See Appendix C for ordering information.

audiotape is mounted. A parent or professional uses the card reader to record a script that the child will say, and when the youngster encounters the card and a photograph in her schedule, she is taught to place the card in the slot in the card reader, listen to the script that is automatically played, and then say the script to a family member or instructor. For example, upon seeing a card and a picture of a tricycle in her schedule, a child might play the script "Watch me," approach a parent and say the script, and then ride the trike. On another page, she might see a card and a picture of a hug, push the button to play the script "I love you," approach a parent and say the script, and receive a hug. Or in response to another page in her schedule, she might approach and say the script, "I did a puzzle." Figure 3-8 shows a card reader and cards. Appendix C provides information about how to purchase them.

After children become proficient schedule followers, and learn to use the pictures, sight words, button-activated recorders, or card readers and cards included in their schedules, these cues can be faded, so that they can independently initiate conversation and select interaction topics and partners. Procedures for fading written and auditory scripts are explained in more detail in Chapter 10 and in *Teaching Conversation to Children with Autism: Scripts and Script Fading* (McClannahan & Krantz, 2005).

If you plan to include the use of a card reader in your child's schedule, it should be placed on a table, desk, or shelf that is easily within reach, and the previously recorded card should be mounted in the schedule book or displayed with the other materials included in the activity schedule.

Lawson

A few weeks after we taught Lawson to accept pennies instead of bites of cookie as rewards for good performance, our other daughter, Cecily, complained that her sister was "stealing" pennies from the cup on her dresser. We were delighted, because it was such concrete evidence that Lawson valued the pennies we were giving her for schedule follow- ing! (We gave Cecily a new coin purse, and helped her find a place for it in a dresser drawer.)

Lewis

Lewis was barely three when we began his photographic activity schedule. In a curriculum catalog, we found some divided wood shelves with heavy-duty plastic containers that fit into each cubby hole. We thought it would be the perfect way to teach him to put his toys away. But he was so small that when he removed a bin from the shelf, he usu- ally dropped it, spilling the contents. He wasn't tall enough to see into the bins, so he made a lot of errors. And when he put the wood puzzle back in the container and attempted to lift it, he often toppled over headfirst because of its weight. We moved that bookcase to his brother's room, and bought shelving that was lower, and clear plastic bins that were lighter and easier for Lewis to manage. Teaching went much faster after the change in bookcases.

Ross

Ross already knew how to vacuum the living room, but he never helped out unless we asked, so we took a picture of him in the living room, holding the handle of the vacuum, and added it to his activity schedule. Every time he turned the page and looked at the picture, he went straight to the candy dish on the coffee table, and we always had to guide him to his schedule. One evening, while we were discussing his progress, we flipped through his schedule book, and suddenly we both noticed that, in the dark background of the photograph, we could see the candy dish. For

Ross, that was the most important part of that picture. We took a new photo the next day, hanging a white sheet behind Ross to achieve a plain background. It took several weeks of teaching to help him avoid this error, because he had practiced it so many times.

4 | A Different Way to Teach

It isn't customary to manually guide children through activities, and it looks a bit strange. Why do we recommend such an unusual teaching procedure? The answer is related to prompts.

Prompts are instructions, gestures, demonstrations, touches, or other things that we arrange or do to increase the likelihood that children will make correct responses. Lovaas (1977) defined a prompt as an event that "cues the desired response prior to training or with minimal training" (p. 20). For example, the teacher says, "Stand up," and if the child does not stand up, the adult lifts him to a standing position. Of course, our goal is to remove prompts as soon as possible, so that children can make correct responses without our help.

In discrete-trial language training, we often prompt children by telling them what to say. ("What's this? Say 'apple'.") Typically, in discrete-trial teaching, the adult gives an instruction or asks a question, the child responds, the adult delivers a reward, the child eats the snack or plays with the toy, and then waits for the next trial to begin. The child's responses are: wait, respond, and use or consume a reward. Thus, passive waiting is one of the responses that is repeatedly rewarded (McClannahan & Krantz, 1997). This may explain why many children with autism who have learned to talk and to do many useful activities do not speak or engage in familiar tasks unless instructed to do so. This is one of the problems that we address when we teach youngsters to follow activity schedules—we teach them to initiate and complete activities and go on to the next activities without waiting for someone to give them directions.

The procedure for teaching activity schedules differs from regular education in another way as well. Teachers of normally developing children usually use a sequence of least-to-most prompts. The teacher asks a question ("Where is your clavicle?") and if the student does not respond, or responds incorrectly, she may model a correct response ("Watch me point to my clavicle"). If the student still does not make a correct response, the teacher may then guide his hand toward his shoulder, and she may even tell him the answer ("Your collarbone is your clavicle").

Although the least-to-most prompts sequence may be successful for typically developing children, it is often ineffective for children with autism, because it permits them to make many errors. After errors occur, they are likely to be repeated, and it becomes increasingly difficult to help a child avoid them. In addition, because we do not deliver rewards for incorrect performances, the child may become inattentive or disruptive.

Why Manual Guidance?

In contrast to the instructional procedures discussed above, the procedure used to teach activity schedules is a most-to-least prompts sequence with manual guidance. We begin with full manual guidance, in order to prevent errors, and we gradually decrease guidance as the child learns the correct responses. The careful reduction of physical guidance is called graduated guidance. Then we move to spatial fading, shadowing, and decreasing our physical proximity, which are discussed later in this chapter. These procedures promote independence and enable young people with autism to complete activities without immediate supervision (Pierce & Schreibman, 1994).

Preparing to Teach

Before the first teaching session, arrange the materials. Place the photographic activity schedule on the far left of the work surface, and then sequence the materials on the work surface, or on nearby shelves from left to right, in the order that they will be used. (Later, when the youngster has acquired more schedule-following skills, it will be important to intermittently rearrange materials, so that he must scan the shelves to find the depicted items.) If you want your child to work or play at a desk

Fig. 4-1 | How to Teach Schedule-Following Skills

PREPARE TO TEACH
- Arrange materials
- Prepare rewards
- Put tokens nearby

GIVE AN INITIAL INSTRUCTION
(e.g., "Please find something to do.")

USE FULL MANUAL GUIDANCE TO
- Open book or turn page
- Point to photograph
- Obtain materials
- Complete activity
- Put materials away

DELIVER REWARDS
- Deliver edibles from behind
- Deliver tokens from behind
- Make delivery of tokens visible

USE PROMPT-FADING PROCEDURES:
- Graduated guidance
- Spatial fading
- Shadowing
- Decreasing physical proximity

USE ERROR-CORRECTION PROCEDURES:
- Return to previous prompt-fading procedure
- Close the schedule book and begin the session again
- Start over; Return to manual guidance and re-teach the entire schedule
- Re-evaluate the power of the rewards
- Substitute a new activity for one that produces many errors

or table, locate it nearby. If he will play on the floor, be sure that there is an open, uncluttered area adjacent to the target materials. Arrange the available space so that the schedule book will always be clearly visible.

If you will use snacks as rewards (for example, bites of cheese, pieces of apple or cookie, grapes, or cereal), put these in a container that will be easy for you to reach. Do not use large bites or snacks that are not quickly consumed (such as caramels, gummy bears, or hard candy) or you may find that your youngster is still enjoying his reward while making an error. If your child has learned to use a token system, place it near him on the work surface.

It will be helpful if you can give the child your undivided attention. For example, try to avoid answering the door or the telephone or carrying on conversations with family members or colleagues during teaching sessions. Don't worry, however, about noise from the television, the sounds of siblings or other students at play, or the occasional entry of another family member or therapist. Youngsters must learn to engage in activities when distractions are present.

The Initial Instruction

When you are ready to begin the teaching session, give the child one initial instruction, such as "Play with your toys," "Find something to do," or "It's time to do your after-school jobs." Select a direction that is quite general, and that will be comfortable and appropriate even after he or she is a proficient schedule follower. You may want to select an instruction that you give to your other children, such as "Go play," or "Please get busy."

Give the initial instruction only once. After you have given it, do not talk to your child again until he turns to a picture that indicates that he should interact with you, or until he has completed his schedule. Remember, you are teaching independence from adult instructions.

Manual Guidance

After giving the initial instruction, step behind your child and guide her to her activity schedule. This is typically accomplished by holding her shoulders or upper arms and moving her toward the schedule. Put your hands over her hands, and help her open the schedule book and point to the first picture. Then guide her to the target materials, and guide her to pick them up and deposit them on the floor or on a nearby work surface.

Next, guide her to complete the task depicted in her schedule book. If it is a familiar task (such as completing a frame-tray puzzle) provide only the amount of guidance needed to prevent errors. When the puzzle is completed, guide her to pick it up and return it to its position on the shelf or work surface. Then guide her back to the schedule, and guide her to turn the page, point to the next picture, obtain relevant materials, take them to the desk or floor, and complete that task.

Repeat this procedure for every activity in the photographic schedule. Manually guide your child to:

1. open the schedule book or turn a page;
2. point to a photograph;
3. obtain the depicted materials and take them to the work area;
4. complete the task;
5. return the materials to their original location; and
6. return to the schedule and turn a page.

Parents and teachers frequently report that the most difficult aspect of this teaching procedure is remembering not to talk to the child. Remind yourself that your verbal instructions may become embedded in the activities, preventing your son or daughter or student from achieving independence.

Delivering Rewards

When you begin to teach schedule following, deliver rewards frequently. If you are using snack foods as rewards, deliver them from behind your child. If he is cooperative and working well, reach around and place a bit of snack food in his mouth. Try to time the delivery of the reward so that it occurs simultaneously with his appropriate behavior. Do this as frequently as possible, but don't reward him if he is delaying, making an error, resisting your guidance, or engaging in tantrum behavior or stereotypy.

Children who have learned to use token systems do not need immediate food rewards. If you are using a token system, give coins, stickers, or happy faces often, and attempt to deliver them in such a way that the youngster will notice them. When he is using his schedule, or obtaining or putting away materials, the token board should be nearby on the work surface, where he can easily see the delivery of tokens. When he is playing on the floor or completing an activity at a desk, move the token board to that location, but remember to deliver tokens from behind him, not from in front, and to deliver them only when he is working appropriately. When mentoring new teachers and therapists, we have noticed that it is helpful to remind them that the behavior a child is displaying when a reward is delivered is a behavior that is likely to increase in frequency. If we reward children at the moment that they are pointing to pictures in their schedules, they will be more likely to point to the pictures. If we reward them at the moment that they are pausing and doing nothing, such delays will be more frequent. Don't reward behavior that you don't want your child to repeat.

Many children who embark on first activity schedules have begun to use token systems, but earn only four or five tokens before these are exchanged for a preferred food or activity. With these children, pennies, stickers, or other types of tokens should be augmented by tangible rewards. For example, you might give your child bites of a snack while he points to a picture and obtains and completes the depicted activity, but give him a token when he puts the materials away. Timing the delivery of the last token with the last activity (such as a special snack) may increase the value of the tokens. Remember that the tokens are exchanged for an additional reward (a special toy, snack, tickle, or play activity, accompanied by your praise and attention).

Some Do's and Don'ts

We have already mentioned one "don't"—don't talk to your youngster while he is learning to follow his schedule, unless the schedule dictates a social activity. You have selected some activities that you want him to do all by himself; help him by curtailing your talk, so that he won't be dependent on your instructions.

Another don't—don't gesture. Ultimately, your child will own his schedule, and will select, sequence, and complete activities on his own. But if your gestures become relevant cues, he won't achieve this level of independence. When in doubt, guide him from behind, but don't point to his schedule book or toys.

When we train novice teachers and therapists, we often tell them, "Stay out of the way." That is, don't place any part of your body between the child and his schedule or materials. The presence of clothing and a picture of clothing in an activity schedule should evoke dressing; an available computer and a picture of a computer in an activity should result in keyboarding; a food preparation task and a picture of hands under the faucet should result in hand washing. Standing between a child and his materials, or reaching in front of rather than behind him, may delay his learning to complete a task independently.

On the other hand, you can make some critical decisions that will promote independence. If a child begins to engage in stereotypic or disruptive behavior, quickly guide him to do the scheduled activity. If he delays in pointing to a picture, obtaining materials, or completing the activity, use manual guidance before he makes an incorrect or inappropriate response. If he cries, verbally objects, or attempts to stop the activity, guide him to continue. Figure 4-2 summarizes some of the do's and don'ts.

Fig. 4-2 | Some Do's and Don'ts about Teaching

DO	DON'T
Display materials on shelf or bookcase	Attempt to teach a first schedule in a cluttered or disorganized environment
Arrange not to answer the door or phone	Worry about noise from TV or other children
Arrange materials in sequence	Get between the child and the materials
Prepare rewards in advance	Use these rewards at other times
Give one initial instruction	Talk, except during social activities
Use manual guidance and guide quickly to prevent errors or delays	Point, gesture, model, or reach in front of the child
Deliver rewards frequently	Deliver rewards when the child is delaying or behaving inappropriately

Graduated Guidance

As noted above, teaching begins with full, hand-over-hand manual guidance. But after a few sessions, you will notice that your child is becoming less dependent upon your guidance. You may feel him move his arm to turn a page, or feel him turn toward the bookshelf, or reach to pick up Lego blocks and put them back in the basket without depending on your help. Try lightly resting your hands on his without guiding. His responses will let you know how much guidance is necessary. For example, if he puts the pieces in the puzzle without your guidance, don't continue to guide. But do use guidance to prevent errors. If you feel his arms reaching for a toy that does not correspond to the photograph in his schedule, immediately guide his hands to the correct toy. If he often attempts to put beads in his mouth, prevent this behavior by guiding him to string the beads.

Typically, children master some tasks quickly, and others more slowly. Some youngsters need sustained manual guidance in order to learn to turn pages; others need continuing guidance to learn to return materials to their original locations on the shelves; still others need ongoing guidance to learn to run cards through the card reader or to push buttons on voice recorders. By carefully attending to your child's movements, you will learn which responses to guide and which responses no longer require your guidance. If you are merely covering his hands with yours while he does the target activity, you are ready to move to spatial fading.

Spatial Fading

Spatial fading means gradually changing the location of manual prompts (Cooper, 1987). If a youngster systematically points to pictures in her schedule, her teacher may stop using hand-over-hand prompts for these tasks, and may now lightly hold her wrist. If she continues to point to the pictures, the teacher may lightly hold her forearm, and later her upper arm and then her elbow. And if correct responding continues, the teacher may eventually only touch her shoulder when she points.

The skillful use of these teaching procedures depends upon careful observation of a child's behavior. When teaching a first schedule, you will no doubt find that you must continue to use graduated guid-

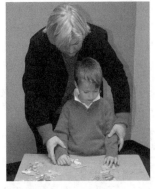

(Fig. 4-3) *(left)* Puzzles were included in several of Jack's previous activity schedules, but he had never assembled one with so many pieces. His instructor used graduated guidance to help him get started.

(below left) When there were pauses that lasted more than ten seconds, she used spatial fading—she touched his upper arms or shoulders.

(below middle) When Jack remained engaged with the activity, his instructor shadowed his movements.

(below right) Then she gradually moved away from him and faded her proximity.

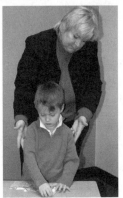 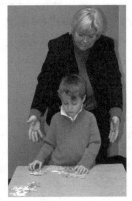 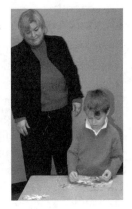

ance for some responses, but that you can use spatial fading for others. Waiting too long to fade prompts slows children's progress, but fading prompts too soon results in errors that also impede learning. You will learn from your child when to fade.

Shadowing

If your child performs the desired behavior when you are merely touching his shoulder, you may begin to shadow him. Shadowing means that you follow his movements very closely with your hands, but without touching him (Cooper, 1987), and if he continues to display correct responses, you gradually move your hands farther away from him.

When Owen was learning to follow his first schedule, we found that he, like most other children with autism, required a combination of graduated guidance, spatial fading, and shadowing. He quickly learned to obtain materials and we were soon shadowing these responses, with the exception that he often attempted to have his snack before opening the schedule book. We continued graduated guidance in order to prevent this error. While manually guiding to prevent him from throwing the stacking cups, we used spatial fading to help him put the shapes in the shape box. Although he learned to complete some tasks more quickly than others, he eventually completed all of them with shadowing, and it was time to increase the distance between him and his teacher.

Decreasing Physical Proximity

When your youngster correctly completes all of the components of the activity schedule with shadowing, take the final prompt-fading step—fade your presence. Initially you may step back and increase the distance between you and your child by six inches. In the next session, if correct responses continue, you may stand one foot away. Like other decisions about prompt fading, decisions about decreasing proximity are based upon your child's performance. If he continues to make correct responses in the next sessions, move one foot away, then two feet away, and so on.

When group home therapists shadowed him, Al, age 10, correctly completed a morning activity schedule that included photographs of getting dressed and making his bed. Next they decreased their distance in six-inch increments. When they were one foot away and Al completed the target activities without errors, they moved eighteen inches away, then two feet away, and so on. Eventually, they stood outside his bedroom door, and then moved around the corner and out of sight. Covert observation and checks of his bedroom and his appearance when he emerged showed that he now dressed and made his bed without immediate supervision.

Dealing with Errors

All children make errors when learning to follow activity schedules. Initially they do not know what is expected of them. In addition, most have previously learned some responses that are incompatible with schedule following, such as waiting for an adult to give an instruction or provide play materials; helping themselves to snacks that are now included in the schedule; repeatedly flipping rather than turning pages of books; or spinning toys, rather than using them for their intended purposes.

The most-to-least prompts sequence, discussed earlier, is designed to prevent errors whenever possible, but even the most expert clinicians are sometimes unable to do this. Occasionally, a child moves with surprising speed, engages in a completely unexpected behavior, successfully evades manual guidance, engages in disruptive behavior, or appears to be making a correct response that, at the last moment, is transformed into an error.

The strategy for dealing with errors is: Return to the previous prompting procedure. If you are shadowing a child who makes an error, return to spatial fading. If you are using spatial fading, return to graduated guidance. And if you are using graduated guidance, return to full, hand-over-hand manual guidance. Continue to use the previous prompting procedure until the youngster has made one or more correct responses on the schedule component associated with the error; then again fade prompts. For example, if the child attempts to move on to the next part of the schedule before putting materials away, return to the previous prompting procedure until he has correctly returned one or two bins to the shelf. If this error occurs near the end of the schedule, it may be necessary to use the prior prompting procedure in the next teaching session.

If you are using graduated guidance and your son tries to obtain materials before turning the page and pointing to the picture of those materials, use full manual guidance to help him turn the page and point to the picture. Continue to use full guidance on the next several opportunities to turn a page and point to the picture, and then return to graduated guidance. If you are shadowing your daughter as she puts a piece in a puzzle, and she attempts to put the puzzle away before completing it, return to spatial fading, but if another error occurs, return to graduated guidance.

Repeated errors indicate that a child has not yet really learned the tasks, or has not yet learned to benefit from the prompting procedures. Under these circumstances, you may consider several alternatives. One of these is to start over—to re-teach the entire schedule, beginning again with hand-over-hand guidance. Another option is to respond to errors by closing the schedule book, returning materials to their original locations, and guiding your child to begin the session again. However, don't require him to do one particular activity several times—he may learn that this task is to be completed more than once.

Another way to deal with errors is to shorten the schedule. It is better for your child to correctly complete a schedule that includes three activities than for him to make multiple errors on a schedule that includes four or five activities. You can always add another activity after he completes the first schedule without errors.

You may also want to reconsider the available rewards. Are there other snacks or toys that your child prefers? Are rewards delivered frequently? And you may want to reassess the activities in the schedule. Is a particular activity always associated with errors? For example, does your youngster typically make errors on a color-sorting task, or on a tracing worksheet? Does he usually line up the Lego blocks, rather than building with them? If one activity usually produces errors, it can be removed and replaced by a different photograph and different materials.

Finally, it may be important to evaluate your child's responses to manual guidance. If he regularly tantrums or resists, it may be necessary to temporarily discontinue the activity schedule, and return to the procedures for teaching him to accept touching and guidance (see Chapter 2).

Putting It All Together

By now, you may be wondering how to do so many things simultaneously (see Figure 4-1 for a flow chart of all of these tasks). You must manually guide your child; put edible rewards in his mouth (if tokens have not yet acquired sufficient value); deliver tokens in such a way that he notices that he has earned a coin or sticker; remember which of his responses require graduated guidance, spatial fading, or shadowing; and be prepared to use an error-correction procedure.

Typically we learn this complex repertoire through practice and through feedback from others. Your child's successes and errors may teach you how to change your behavior in the next session. And if you and another person are jointly undertaking this project, you may help one another by observing and commenting on the effective use of the teaching procedures, and on occasions when the teaching procedures were not followed, or were followed inconsistently. Your partner, like your youngster, will be more responsive if rewards such as praise and empathy are more frequent than correction.

Occasionally, both parents and professionals observe that they have inadvertently taught incorrect responses. When this happens, we can take comfort in the scientific knowledge that children's behavior is pliable and responsive to the environment. By changing the teaching procedures, enhancing the rewards, or altering photographs or materials, we can correct errors and help children achieve important next steps.

5 | Measuring Schedule Following

Introduction

Although collecting data is a critical part of teaching a child to use an activity schedule, some parents and teachers are uninterested in it. Teaching a child to follow a schedule requires that you attend to a plethora of details. And when he independently follows the schedule, his new skills will be obvious to you and others. Thus, you may wonder why you should bother with data collection.

There are several answers to this question. First, data on your child's performance will help you identify tasks that are often associated with errors, so that you can be prepared to use the error-correction procedures described in the previous chapter. Second, the data will help you make decisions about when to fade prompts. And finally, the data will reveal when it is time to introduce variations in the schedule, or introduce a new schedule. Although Kip's parents reported that he had mastered his first schedule, data collected by his instructor indicated that he was correctly completing 68% to 74% of schedule components. The data showed that he needed continued teaching in order to achieve success.

Casual observation is often inaccurate. Adults sometimes inadvertently prompt children. For example, taking a small step toward a boy who is about to turn a page, moving a hand toward the toys he should pick up, quickly inhaling when he reaches for the correct materials—these prompts may become more relevant to a youngster than the pictures in his schedule and the corresponding materials. As a result, when such prompts are absent, errors occur.

Collecting Data

Gathering data on a child's use of her schedule isn't really daunting, and it gives us a detailed picture of performance. It allows us to examine many separate responses, and makes it possible to determine which parts of a task are difficult, so that we can be prepared to provide instruction exactly when it is most needed. In order to get this fine-grained analysis of a youngster's schedule-following skills, we break each task into several separate components.

Most activities in the schedule have five components: 1) opening the schedule book or turning a page; 2) looking at and pointing to a picture; 3) obtaining the depicted materials; 4) completing the activity; and 5) putting the materials away. Correct responses are scored plus (+) and incorrect responses are scored minus (–). Before you begin to teach, write the activities in the left column of the data sheet, in the order that they appear in the schedule, and put the data sheet on a clipboard (see Appendix D for a blank data sheet).

Suppose that you are teaching a preschooler to use a six-page schedule book, and the photographs included in the book show a puzzle, a shape box, the youngster being tickled, a Potato Head toy, a color matching task, and raisins on a plate. The first component of the puzzle activity is scored as correct if the youngster opens her schedule book to the first page without any help (see Figure 5-1). The second component, pointing to and looking at the picture, is scored as correct only if she points and looks. Because you are standing behind her, you can't see her eyes, but consider that she is looking if her head is oriented toward the picture. If she is turned away from the picture, gently guide her shoulders to help her orient, and score this component incorrect.

The third component, obtaining materials, is scored as correct if she moves from the schedule to the puzzle or puzzle container, picks it up, and takes it to the work surface or floor. The fourth component, completing the activity, is scored as correct if she puts all of the pieces in the puzzle (and returns the puzzle to the container, if you have provided one). And the fifth component is scored as correct if she returns the puzzle (or puzzle in container) to its original location on the shelf or bookcase.

Fig. 5-1 | Schedule Following Data Sheet

Observer: Dad
Date: December 20, 2009

Activity	Opens Book/Turns page	Points/ Looks	Obtains	Completes	Puts Away
Puzzle	–	+	–	–	–
Shape Box	–	–	+	+	–
Ask for tickle	+	–	N/A	+	N/A
Potato Head	–	–	–	–	–
Color Matching	–	+	–	+	–
Snack	–	+	–	+	–
# Completed	1	3	1	4	0

Number of components correctly completed: 9
Total number of components: 28
Percentage of components correctly completed: 32%

(Fig. 5-1) Sample data sheet used to measure a child's acquisition of schedule-following skills. (Blank data sheets are found in Appendix D.)

Each component is scored as correct only if the child completes it without any help from you. That is, you do not touch her, talk to her, gesture to materials, or do anything else that may assist her in making a correct response. If you provide help of any kind, score that component incorrect. In addition, if the child pauses or delays for more than 10 seconds, or engages in inappropriate behavior, score the component incorrect and prompt a correct response.

Although most activities in the schedule have five components, a few have fewer than five; often, social interaction has only three.

The schedule referenced in Figure 5-1 includes asking for a tickle. The child's tasks are: turn the page, look at and point to the picture of being tickled, go to someone and say "Tickle, please." There are no materials to obtain or put away, and these activity components are scored "NA" (not applicable).

The data sheet in Figure 5-1 shows that the youngster did not independently turn the page to the color-matching picture, and this was scored minus. However, after being guided to turn the page, she did point to and look at the picture of the color-matching materials, and her parent marked a plus for that task component. She needed help in obtaining the color-matching bin, and minus was scored. Although she correctly completed the color-matching task by sticking the red circle on the corresponding red circle, the yellow circle on the yellow circle, and so on, she did not put the materials away until she was prompted to do so, and "puts away" was scored minus.

Having a snack is the final activity shown in Figure 5-1. The schedule included a picture of raisins on a paper plate, and the plate of raisins was displayed on a shelf. The child ate some of the raisins without prompts (her parents did not require that she eat them all), and the activity was scored as correctly completed. She did not put the paper plate in the wastebasket without help, and "putting away" was scored as incorrect.

After a teaching session, add the pluses in each column of the data sheet and enter the totals in the bottom row. This is a good time to review each task component and plan prompting and prompt-fading strategies for the next session.

Next, summarize the data by filling in the blanks at the bottom of the data sheet. Count the total number of components correctly completed, and the total number of components in the schedule. Then divide the number correct by the total number of components and multiply by 100 to obtain the percentage of components correctly completed. In Figure 5-1, 9 of 28 schedule components were scored as correctly completed. The youngster's parents divided 9 by 28 and then multiplied by 100 to obtain the percentage correct (32%). Later in this chapter, we explain how to use this percentage to create a graph that displays a youngster's acquisition of schedule-following skills.

When a child uses a written rather than a photographic activity schedule such as the one described above, the same data-collection procedures apply, but instead of turning a page, the youngster returns to her schedule and makes a checkmark next to the words that describe the activity just completed, or moves a marker to the next activity in the schedule.

Solving Data-Collection Problems

Often one parent teaches schedule following while the other is at work, commuting, attending to other children, preparing meals, shopping, or doing other essential tasks. How can you collect data on your child's performance while using manual guidance and delivering snacks and tokens? The use of a tape recorder is one solution. Turn the recorder on and place it nearby before beginning the session, and record your narration of the outcome of each task component. For example, "Potato Head. Turns page, plus. Points and looks, minus." At a less busy time, you can transcribe this information onto the data sheet.

Some parents invite another child in the family to assist with data collection. Teenagers, and even younger children, may enjoy observing sessions and recording the symbols that you dictate. If you enlist a child's help, teach him or her to stay nearby, and to hold the data sheet where you can see it, so that you can verify correct scoring and indicate when corrections are needed.

Attempting to memorize the data and record them after the session ends is not a good solution to data-collection problems. Few of us can accurately recall twenty or more separate responses and whether they were prompted or unprompted. If you cannot use a tape recorder or enlist the help of your spouse or another child, you may want to withdraw your prompts for a few seconds, or use manual guidance to stop the activity for a few seconds, while you quickly record a plus or minus. Data collection will become much easier as you practice, and as your youngster acquires skills. When you begin to use shadowing, and when you later decrease your proximity, you'll have much more time to record data.

Occasionally you and your partner may be able to collect data at the same time. This exercise can be especially useful if, after the session, you compare your data sheets and talk about agreements and disagreements. These discussions often reveal error patterns or unintended prompts that were not obvious to the person who delivered instruction.

Graphing the Data

A graph gives you a session-to-session, week-to-week, and month-to-month overview of a youngster's acquisition of schedule-following skills. Although you may want to keep and periodically review the data sheets in order to look for error patterns, graphs will be more helpful in tracking a child's overall progress.

On graph paper divided by tens, number the left side of the graph from ten to one hundred, and label it "Percentage of components correctly completed." Label the bottom of the graph "Sessions," and add a date each time you graph another session. If you conduct more than one session per day, you may want to indicate both date and time. At the top of the page, you may add information that will be useful in making later comparisons. For example, "Schedule 1: Puzzle, Pegs, Tickle, Picture Matching, and Corn Chips" (see Figure 5-2).

After each session, add a data point; if the child scored 30% correct, plot 30% on the graph. Experienced clinicians know that graph-

Fig. 5-2 | Photographic Activity Schedule

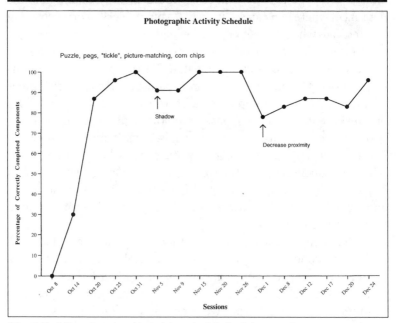

(Fig. 5-2) A first photographic activity schedule for Brice, age 3.

ing is relatively effortless if it is accomplished each day, but becomes drudgery if ungraphed data accumulate. In addition, each day's data point is a bit of information that may be useful in planning the next day's teaching. You can use arrows on graphs to highlight noteworthy events, such as the beginning of shadowing or decreasing proximity (Figure 5-2). You can also use arrows to indicate other changes, such as replacing a photograph or an activity that produced many errors.

One of the most important things to do with a graph is to display it. Show your graph to your son's grandparents, aunts and uncles, and teachers; show it to family friends, and discuss his progress. Just as he needs rewards for learning to follow his schedule, you also need rewards for your hard work in helping him acquire these important skills.

6 | The First Schedule is Mastered!

Introduction

After several consecutive sessions in which your child or student scores 80% to 100% correct, while you are standing eight or ten feet away, you may consider the first schedule mastered. Don't wait too long to take the next steps (described below)—the young person's performance may decline if the same tasks are presented again and again in the same order.

New Activity Sequences

Becoming a schedule follower does not mean learning a specific chain of responses. To be truly independent, children must become "picture readers"—they must learn to do any activity represented by a picture or word in a schedule book. Changing the order of pictures teaches them to attend to and act on cues in the schedule.

Perry was seven when he began his first schedule, which included the following sequence of activities: putting twenty-five pieces in their correct places in the shape-matching game Perfection; drawing a picture, using a stencil and crayon; asking a parent for a "high-five"; sorting pictures of food and clothing into separate containers; and having a snack (popcorn) and putting the paper plate in a nearby wastebasket.

After Perry learned to complete these activities while a parent stood in the doorway of his room and did not prompt, the photographs in his schedule were rearranged. The picture of the Perfection game continued to be first, because his parents were concerned that he would not begin the schedule if a different picture appeared on page one. The picture of popcorn remained on the last page, as a reward for completing the scheduled activities. The other three pictures in his schedule book were placed in a new order—sorting, stencil, and "high five." To help Perry master the new activity sequence, the materials on his shelves were also rearranged, so that the order of the materials matched the order of photographs in his schedule.

On the first teaching session after the photographs were rearranged, Perry independently began his schedule as usual, and completed the Perfection game activity without prompts, after which his father delivered a token by placing it on Perry's nearby clipboard. Upon turning to the second page and encountering a different photograph, the boy stopped for a few seconds, and then rapidly turned pages. At this point, his father quickly stepped forward and manually guided him to point to the picture on page two, obtain the sorting materials, and begin the task. After this prompt to begin, Perry independently completed the sorting activity, put the materials away, and earned another token. He returned to his schedule, turned the page, and again encountered a photograph in a new position. He scrutinized the picture of the crayon and stencil for a full ten seconds, but when his father stepped forward to provide manual guidance, he turned and obtained the materials without help, completed the activity, and put the materials back on the shelf. Because Perry's father prompted him by increasing his proximity, he scored "obtains" as incorrect, but because the revised schedule was unfamiliar and because it wasn't necessary to touch or guide, he placed another token on the token board.

Upon returning to the schedule, turning the page, and again finding a photograph in a new order, Perry darted toward the snack. His father, who had been shadowing, intercepted him, guided him back to the book, and used hand-over-hand guidance to help him point to the picture of "high five." Because Perry vocally objected and engaged in stereotypic arm tensing and finger play, he was guided to give a "high five" (his father participated in this social activity by enthusiastically saying "Yeah, Little Guy!" but did not deliver a token). Subsequently, Perry independently walked back to the book, pointed to the picture of

Fig. 6-1 | Photographic Activity Schedule

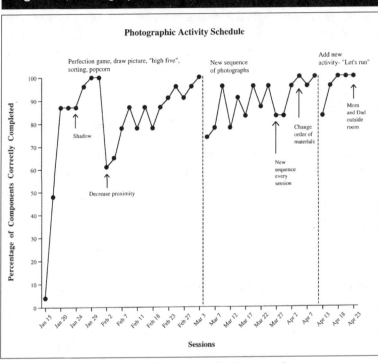

(Fig. 6-1) A first photographic activity schedule for Perry, age 7.

the snack, ate the popcorn, threw away the paper plate, and received his last two tokens, which were exchanged for a roughhousing and tickling game known to his family as "sack the quarterback."

In subsequent sessions, Perry's performance was variable, and his parents continued to shadow him, occasionally providing manual guidance or spatial fading to prevent errors. He began the fifth session by opening the book and examining all of the pages before turning back to page one and pointing to the first picture. Because his perusal was completed in less than ten seconds, he was not prompted. His parents interpreted this as an exploratory response—he appeared to be reviewing the new sequence of photographs.

When Perry's pictures and activities were resequenced, his parents drew a horizontal, dotted line on the graph, and labeled it "New Sequence of Photographs" (see Figure 6-1). When his performance stabilized—he correctly completed 80% to 100% of schedule components without prompts in five consecutive sessions—his mom and dad provided a different sequence of photographs in *each* session and, later, they placed materials on the shelves in an order that did not match the order of pictures in the schedule (see arrows, Figure 6-1). At this time, Perry's parents noted that when they were in his room, he often took their hands and pulled them toward his schedule book, or independently picked it up, opened it, and began to do depicted activities.

Perry's story offers a good example of how to resequence photographs and activities. First, change the order of a few pictures in the schedule, and change the arrangement of materials to match the new picture sequence. Then teach the new sequence until it is mastered. Secondly, rearrange photographs every session, and change the order of all of the pictures. And finally, after performance stabilizes, rearrange materials so that they are no longer presented in an order that matches the sequence of pictures in the schedule book.

New Pictures and Activities

When a child has learned to follow a schedule in which pictures and activities are regularly resequenced, it is time to add a new photograph and activity to his first schedule. You can facilitate the youngster's mastery if you select an activity that is both familiar and preferred. For example, if the last picture in the schedule shows potato chips, you may decide to move this photo to a middle page, and add a new last page that depicts a different but equally rewarding activity, such as juice, a swing in the air, a ride in the wagon, or an opportunity to watch part of a favorite video.

When the new activity is added, be prepared to return to hand-over-hand guidance to help the youngster master the expanded schedule, and use the prompt-fading procedures discussed in Chapter 4 (graduated guidance, spatial fading, shadowing, and decreasing proximity). Perry's parents added his popcorn snack to the first half of his schedule, and added a new, familiar activity, requesting a run around the recreation room, as the sixth and last activity (see Figure 6-1). They also added a sixth token to his token board.

After the first new activity is mastered, add a second new photo to the schedule book, but retain an especially enjoyable activity as the last activity. As in the previous examples, assist your child by selecting a familiar task. Perry's parents added a Lincoln Logs fort as a second new activity; he had previously built the fort with assistance. The photograph in his schedule showed the completed structure, and prompts and prompt-fading procedures enabled him to independently assemble it.

Continue to add new pictures and activities to the schedule, but fit the schedule to your child's capabilities. A preschooler may learn to complete a series of activities that takes about fifteen minutes, but an eight-year-old may engage in scheduled activities for thirty minutes or more. Don't forget to add tokens or other rewards as you add new activities!

New Independence

It's time to emphasize independence after a youngster can complete scheduled activities without assistance when photographs are regularly resequenced, when two or three new activities have been added, and when the materials are frequently rearranged. Return to the procedures detailed in Chapter 4 to decrease your proximity, but continue until you are outside the room and no longer in sight.

Initially you will want to peek in about every 15 seconds, and if your child is not following the schedule, return to the prior prompting procedure (shadowing). But again fade your presence as soon as his performance is stable. If you observe that he is dependably following the schedule, gradually increase the time between observations. Check on him every 30 seconds, then every minute, then every 2 minutes, and so on, until you are doing only a few random, unpredictable observations.

If you have been giving your child tokens for schedule following, you will want to decrease the frequency of token delivery at the same time that you fade your presence. Instead of giving your youngster one token at a time, give him two or three tokens when you make occasional checks, provide the last tokens after he has finished the schedule, and immediately let him exchange the tokens for the special activity. Independence grows and develops when it is systematically rewarded. It is important to increase the amount of reinforcement as you decrease your proximity.

At this point, you will have created a ten- to thirty-minute period during which you can turn your attention to other matters, such as finishing the laundry, starting dinner preparation, helping another child with homework, or enjoying a well-deserved coffee break. But at regular intervals—for example, every third session, or every fifth session—you'll still want to observe continuously and collect data. The data will alert you to problems that can often be corrected in a few sessions, using the original teaching procedures.

New Problems, Familiar Solutions

The last step in prompt fading—fading the adult's proximity—is often the most difficult. It's not unusual for children to make errors or engage in stereotypy when parents or teachers are no longer in sight. Although some youngsters perform as well as before when adults are no longer visible, others must have more exposure to the prompt-fading procedures, especially the last procedure—decreasing proximity. *The absence of adults is the ultimate test of whether we have diminished the prompt dependence discussed in Chapter 1.*

If returning to the prior prompting procedure does not resolve a child's performance problems, consider some alternate strategies. One of these is to step in when the first error occurs, and use full manual guidance for the remainder of the session. On the next session, resume fading of proximity, but be prepared to return to manual guidance if the child makes an error. The data on schedule following will reveal whether this tactic is effective; if it achieves the desired outcome, the youngster's percentage correct will gradually increase over several sessions.

If returning to manual guidance for the remainder of the session does not achieve the desired result, explore another alternative. Step in when the first error occurs, put materials away, and close the schedule book. Then guide the child to start the schedule from the beginning, and use hand-over-hand manual guidance for the entire session. At the next opportunity for schedule following, return to fading your proximity but close the schedule book, start over, and use full manual guidance if an error is again observed.

Another option, which provides children with very clear feedback, is token removal, sometimes called response cost (Lutzker, Mc-Gimsey-McRae, & McGimsey, 1983, p.42). Take away a token when the youngster makes an error, and return it when he is performing well.

If errors persist over several sessions, take tokens but do not return them, and allow the child to learn that if he has not earned all of the tokens, he cannot exchange them for a special activity or treat. You may also decide to take away tokens in addition to providing manual guidance (described above).

If none of these strategies is effective, return to the prompts (graduated guidance, spatial fading, shadowing) that enable your child to be successful and repeat the prompt-fading procedures, but this time, fade prompts more slowly. It may be especially important to do more gradual fading of your physical proximity. You might try increasing your distance six inches at a time. Although it may take a considerable amount of time to fade your proximity, remember the importance of this endeavor—it can help your child achieve real independence.

When exploring solutions to new problems, parents and teachers often find it helpful to review their own behavior. The following points are especially important:

- Verbal instructions and gestures should not be used to teach schedule-following skills.
- Prompts should be used to prevent errors whenever possible.
- When errors are corrected or tokens are removed, adults should be nonemotional and matter-of-fact.
- Correct responses should be rewarded immediately with tokens or edibles.
- Young people should receive special attention and preferred activities after completing their schedules.

Finally, regular data-collection and graphing is essential to problem solving. Your data will tell you whether you have helped your child surmount performance problems.

New Schedules

If your child follows a schedule without your help (although you may be just beyond the doorway, or at the other end of a large room), it's time to consider adding a new schedule. But don't abandon the first one. Continue to resequence the pictures and materials and continue to reward correct performance.

Occasionally you may also remove a photograph and a corresponding task from the first schedule, and replace an old activity with a new one, to add interest. Over a period of time, the activities you remove can be used to construct a second schedule—one that can be packaged in a book bag or backpack and completed at grandma's house, on a family vacation, or during a time of day that is particularly busy.

In addition to creating a new schedule from old activities, push on to new territory. Your youngster's schedule-following skills will grow as a result of each new schedule that is mastered. As a parent of a child with autism, you are probably very busy and over-committed. This is a good time to consider how the next schedule can make a positive contribution to family life. For example, if your daughter completes her schedule in ten minutes, but you need twenty minutes per school day to help her older sibling with homework, create a new schedule comprised of activities that are similar to those in previous schedules. For example, include a different shape box and a different set of stacking toys, replace a five-piece puzzle with a six-piece puzzle, and substitute animal crackers for Teddy Graham crackers.

If morning is a particularly hectic time, you may want to develop a new schedule that facilitates completion of morning routines. Such a schedule might include pictures that cue a preschooler to put her cereal bowl and juice glass on the counter after breakfast, put her book bag and coat near the front door, and obtain and use "See "N" Say" toys until the bus arrives.

For an older child, a morning schedule might include obtaining a glass and bowl, pouring juice and cereal, eating breakfast, putting a lunchbox in a book bag, putting the book bag near the front door, and watching television until the bus arrives. As your child becomes a more proficient schedule follower, you can make decisions about whether to add new activities that are familiar and previously mastered, or activities that your youngsters hasn't yet learned to do. If he doesn't yet know how to put his lunchbox in his book bag, you'll have to manually guide these responses initially, and later fade your prompts. Although it's a busy time of day, the lunchbox has to end up in the book bag, and the morning routine will eventually run more smoothly if your son learns to do these tasks himself.

Some youngsters with autism tantrum when family routines are altered. Consider developing a schedule that will help your child deal with change. You might begin with a schedule book that includes photographs of a familiar play activity; obtaining hat and coat; saying "Let's go," or taking your hand; walking with you to the mailbox; and returning to the house for a snack. When this schedule is mastered, replace getting the mail with riding a trike, and later, with going to the convenience store, bringing in the garbage cans, transporting a sibling, or picking up a commuting parent at the train or bus station. The goal is to rotate these activities as needed to accommodate family members' schedules.

Initially each new activity schedule will require the same (or almost the same) effort and attention to detail that was necessary to teach the first schedule. But if you are systematic in teaching schedule following, this investment will eventually yield important benefits for your child with autism and other members of your family, and later schedules will be mastered more quickly.

7 | When Do Activities End?

Introduction

The activities discussed in previous chapters all have clear endings. The stacking rings are completed when all rings are on the spindle, a worksheet is finished when each item has been answered, and a social activity is over after the youngster initiates and someone responds. But some activities are of indeterminate length, and many children who are successful schedule-followers have not yet learned to tell time. How long should a child watch television, play with dolls or cars, or play computer games?

Using Timers

Many young people who have learned to follow photographic activity schedules quickly learn to set timers, if we teach these skills within the already-familiar context of schedule following. Setting an inexpensive digital kitchen timer typically requires only a few button presses, and photographs in the youngster's schedule can cue these responses.

Small electronic timers are available in hardware and variety stores. Timers with magnets on the back are particularly convenient, because they can be easily mounted on the clipboard used for delivering tokens. These timers often have buttons of different colors, and it is therefore possible to add pictorial cues to the activity schedule to teach a child to press the buttons in a particular sequence.

Suppose that a five-year-old nonreader enjoys looking at picture books, and we want to add this activity to her schedule. We observe that she often looks at books for three to five minutes before losing interest, and we decide to teach her to set a timer for three minutes. This requires pushing the "clear" button once, pushing the "min" button three times, and pushing the "start" button once.

The activity schedule displays a picture of the timer, which cues the child to remove it from her clipboard; next, it highlights the black clear button (which she will press once), three pictures of the white minute button (which she will push three times), and one picture of the red start button (which she will push once). This sequence of pictures is shown in Figure 7-1. If the timer does not have different-colored keys, we can modify it, using small pieces of colored plastic tape.

The teaching procedures are familiar. When the child first encounters the new pictures in her schedule, we use manual guidance to help her point to a photograph of the timer; pick it up and place it on a work surface; point to the picture of the black key and press that key; point to the picture of the white key and press it; and so on. When the timer rings, we immediately guide her to put the books away, return to the schedule, turn the page, and continue. Just as before, graduated guidance is replaced by spatial fading, shadowing, and then decreasing proximity. And just as before, attempts to complete new tasks are followed by rewards even though they are prompted, but as soon as possible, rewards are delivered only for unprompted responses.

Learning to use timers creates new options for many children. Jerry, age 7, liked to draw, and often drew pictures for extended periods, meanwhile neglecting other tasks. He learned to set a timer for ten minutes and move on to the next activity when drawing time ended. Duncan, age 10, enjoyed playing an electronic keyboard; the timer signaled him when it was time to do something else. Thirteen-year-old Vic was a connoisseur of *Star Trek* videos. Because he had acquired some arithmetic skills, his schedule showed a numeral beside a picture of the minute button, and his parents frequently changed the number of minutes of viewing time, so that Vic's schedule would be compatible with other family members' schedules.

After learning to use timers, many children (including those without math skills) begin to "cheat." They set the timer for less than

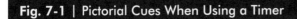

Fig. 7-1 | Pictorial Cues When Using a Timer

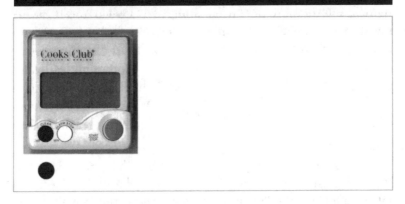

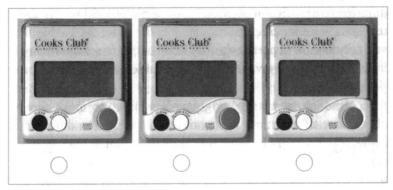

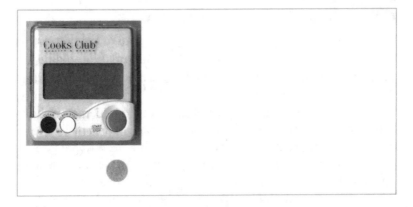

(Fig. 7-1) Pictorial cues used to help a child learn to set a timer. Initially, each picture appears on a separate page of the schedule book.

the specified amount of time when doing less-preferred activities, and for more time when doing favorite activities. "Cheating" often means that it is time to offer choices. Youngsters who read may be ready for a textual cue such as, "Set timer—my choice." Nonreaders may be given similar opportunities by replacing a number in the schedule with a blank space.

Many children with autism engage in repetitive or dysfunctional behavior if an activity lasts too long. When teaching children to make choices about how to allot time, do not use manual guidance if the child sets the timer for an appropriate amount of time, but guide the youngster if he or she attempts to select an amount of time that is much longer or shorter than the desirable duration of a particular activity. For example, if a girl who is about to watch *Sesame Street* videos sets the timer for 15 minutes, you may decide to permit this; if she attempts to set the timer for 50 minutes, you may want to manually guide her to select a shorter period of time.

Although we want young people to learn to make choices about how to use time, we continue to specify the duration of some activities. If the schedule indicates that typing practice should last 10 minutes and your son sets the timer for 5 minutes, use the error-correction procedures discussed in Chapters 4 and 6. Learning to make choices is important, but following parents' and teachers' instructions is equally important!

Other Time-Management Skills

After learning to use a digital timer, a child may quickly learn to set a microwave oven. Many children enjoy activity schedules that teach them to use a microwave oven to make popcorn, or to heat muffins, pretzels, tortillas, or other snacks. In constructing such a schedule, include photographs of each part of the activity—for example, pictures that cue getting the microwave popcorn bag and a bowl from the cupboard, putting popcorn in the oven, pressing the relevant keys on the microwave key pad, removing the popcorn when the timer rings, opening the popcorn bag, and pouring popcorn into a bowl.

Although your child may appear interested in the popcorn (or other snack depicted in his schedule) remember that correct schedule-following responses should be followed by tokens or other tangible rewards. And when the schedule is completed and the snack is ready to eat, you may increase the power of this reward by arranging for the youngster to consume the snack outdoors at the picnic table, or in front of a favorite DVD or TV program.

Pictures that cue setting the microwave are similar to the pictures used to teach setting a kitchen timer. For example, the schedule might show separate pictures of the microwave key pad that highlight the "time cook," "4," "min," and " start" keys. If the child does not yet read, use plastic tape to color-code the microwave key pad and the pictures in the schedule book, so that he can match the pictures to the key pad.

After learning to use activity schedules and timers, some young people learn more sophisticated food preparation tasks. Patrick learned to make brownies and bake them in an electric oven. His schedule displayed all of the relevant steps, including setting the correct oven temperature and putting on arm-length oven mitts before using the oven. Because it was difficult for him to determine when the dough was adequately mixed, he set a kitchen timer for 3 minutes, and continued to stir for that period of time. After putting the brownies in the oven, his schedule cued him to set the timer again and clip it to his belt; when the alarm sounded, he returned to the kitchen, put on the oven mitts, and removed the brownies from the oven.

Walt, age 16, used a photographic schedule to make a meatloaf dinner. Initially, using the activity schedule, he learned to make only the meatloaf. After this was mastered, his schedule was expanded to include making a salad, then preparing a frozen vegetable, and finally, warming dinner rolls. Subsequently he learned to make a spaghetti dinner, and his food preparation skills continue to expand. Time-management skills for adolescents and adults are discussed in more detail in Chapter 11.

Time-Management Skills and Family Life

After your child learns to use timers, consider how these skills may contribute to your family's routines. If there is a safe outdoor area for jogging, biking, or shooting baskets, you may decide to include time in your child's schedule for these activities. If you are computer users, include time for playing computer games (with manual guidance, many youngsters readily learn to use a mouse, and to open and close preferred programs). If your son is a "couch potato," use his schedule to establish times for watching television. If your daughter resists getting out of the tub, use a timer to establish a predictable end of bathtime as part of a going-to-bed or bathtime activity schedule.

Don't forget to teach your child to set timers for varying amounts of time. At grandma's house, there may be more time for watching television. If company is expected, both computer use and bath time may need to be abbreviated. If we frequently allocate different amounts of time for the activities in children's schedules, they are less likely to resist schedule changes that must be made because of family commitments or unexpected events.

8 | Increasing Choice

Introduction

Dealing with unstructured time is difficult for many young people with autism. When parents or instructors do not provide activities, some youngsters do nothing at all, and others display disruptive or stereotypic behavior. Teaching your child to make choices among activities is an important step toward helping him or her learn to make productive use of time, and photographic activity schedules can help.

Teaching Children to Choose Rewards

Almost all youngsters can learn to make choices if we provide an appropriate program of instruction. Your child's initial schedules included pictures of preferred snacks, toys, or activities, such as a cup of yogurt, a piggy-back ride, a drink of juice, or blowing bubbles. The next task is to teach him to choose one of two rewards.

Display the photographs that represent available choices on a large foam board or bulletin board. Select two familiar pictures of "special" or preferred activities, place these photographs in baseball card holders, attach them to the board with Velcro, and place this "choice board" on a shelf or work surface that is easily seen by your youngster. For example, when he was a preschooler, the first two photographs mounted on Tod's choice board were Cheerios and a rocking horse.

The next step is to add a blank page to your child's activity schedule book (this page displays only a Velcro dot). Then invite your child to follow his schedule as usual, but be prepared to prompt. When he turns to the blank page, manually guide him to point to the Velcro dot, go to the choice board, select one of the two photographs, mount it in his schedule book, and then do the activity he selected. As he learns to do this sequence, use the previously described prompt-fading procedures.

Rapid fading of prompts is especially important when the youngster is standing in front of the choice board and oriented toward the two photographs. Guide his arm so that his hand is equidistant from the two pictures and then wait to see if he will make a selection. If he doesn't immediately choose a picture, continue to wait as long as possible, but guide him to make a choice before he begins to engage in off-task or inappropriate behavior. On each subsequent opportunity for choice making, continue to delay your manual guidance and wait to see whether he will reach for a photograph, but use guidance as needed to prevent errors. Remember not to use verbal prompts such as "Choose one" or "Take a picture," because this may teach the child to wait for your instructions rather than to make independent choices.

After your son has learned to choose one of two activities from the choice board, add a third picture, then a fourth, and so on. When he has learned to select from a field of three to five photographs that depict activity choices, add a second blank page to his schedule.

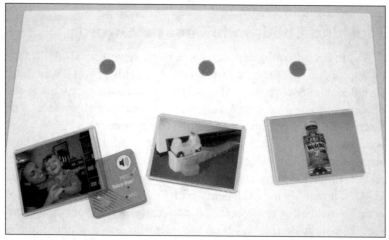

(Fig. 8-1) A choice board that displays three choices.

Over time, continue to add new pictures to the choice board that show other special snacks, toys, or social games that your son enjoys. As the choices expand, you may decide to rotate the pictures on a daily basis. Removing some pictures and adding others makes the choice board more interesting. And don't forget to continue your son's token system—give him coins for making choices, as well as for following the other parts of his schedule. After he finishes his schedule, help him exchange his tokens for an extra-special activity.

Sherman

When he was 32 months old, Sherman mastered his first schedule, which included five photographs. Pictures were resequenced, then new pictures were added, and then a choice was introduced. He had recently conquered a variety of matching tasks, and often took our hands and pulled us toward those materials, so we included a shape-matching task as one of his choices. The other choice was a favorite snack, animal crackers. He quickly learned to select a photograph, put it in his book, and do the pictured activity, but he almost always chose matching, and rarely selected snack. When we introduced a second blank page and a second opportunity to choose, we added a photograph of a number-matching activity. Then he began to vary his choice of matching tasks, and often selected animal crackers when he encountered the second blank page.

Paula

Paula, now 10 years old, learned to follow a photographic schedule three years ago, and presently chooses from a large array of photographs displayed on a choice board. Her choices include playing several different computer games; watching segments of different videos; playing an electronic keyboard; using headphones to listen to music; preparing and eating snacks (for example, cheese and crackers, celery sticks filled with cream cheese, or bread and jelly); looking at books and magazines; playing card games (Uno and Slap Jack) with family members or peers; shooting baskets; and riding her bike. She sets a digital timer for specified amounts of time, and returns to her schedule when the timer rings. Frequent changes in the pictures displayed on her choice board appear to heighten her interest and promote conversation.

Teaching Children to Sequence Their Own Activities

After children have learned to select preferred activities, it is time to teach them to build their own schedules. We adults make ongoing decisions about what to do first and next. We may decide that, after attending to daily housekeeping chores and doing the laundry, we will do something more interesting, such as telephoning a relative or shopping for clothing. At work, we may review a boring report before beginning a more creative task. And sometimes, we avoid less-preferred jobs as long as possible; we weed a flower bed, get the mail, surf the internet, and read a new magazine before doing the dishes and taking out the garbage. These decisions have an impact on the quality of day-to-day life.

Similarly, we can enhance the quality of life for young people with autism by teaching them to sequence their own activities. A child who selects reward activities from a choice board can also learn to select and sequence required activities.

To help a child learn this skill, remove the photographs from the schedule book and attach them (with Velcro) to the inside front and back covers of a new three-ring binder of a different color. Then add one or more new pages to the schedule book to represent reward choices. If your child is a reader, the new pages may display the words "My choice"; if she does not yet read, display a photograph of the choice board.

Once again use graduated guidance, spatial fading, shadowing, and decreased proximity to help your daughter learn to open her new three-ring binder, select a photograph, mount the picture in her schedule book, obtain the materials, complete the activity, put materials away, return to her schedule book, turn the page, and open her new notebook to select a photograph of the next activity. When she is about to select a picture, use only the amount of manual guidance necessary to prevent errors. Minimal guidance will help her learn to choose.

At age four, Libby learned to sequence ten preschool activities. Photographs of preacademic, language, and leisure activities were mounted on the inside covers of a red binder. She selected a photograph from the red notebook, attached it to a page of her blue schedule book, obtained the necessary materials, completed the activity (sometimes with instruction from her teacher), put the materials away, and selected a different photograph. Pictures of her choice board in

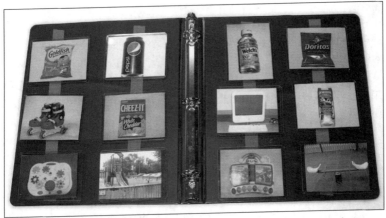

(Fig. 8-2) A choice book for a 7-year-old who has learned to make many choices.

the blue schedule book cued her to select a picture from her choice board, attach it to the same page, and engage in a preferred activity. Her choice board included photographs of a slide, a hippety hop ball, jello, balloons, and a top.

The number of opportunities to select rewards should reflect your child's current schedule-following skills. If your daughter recently completed a seven-page activity schedule in which the third and seventh pages presented opportunities to select a preferred activity, continue this schedule while you teach her to sequence her learning activities. And continue to deliver tokens that are exchanged for a special treat when the schedule is completed.

All of us appreciate choice-making opportunities. Research shows that when people with developmental disabilities learn to choose the order of their activities, their appropriate engagement with assigned tasks increases (Anderson, Sherman, Sheldon, and McAdam, 1997). In addition, when prompts are faded, time on task remains high (Watanabe and Sturmey, 2003). Learning to sequence daily activities is another step toward independence.

Teaching Children to Deliver Their Own Rewards

When your child consistently sequences his required activities and chooses among several preferred activities, teach him to deliver his own tokens. To accomplish this objective, attach the tokens or coins to the bottom of every page in his schedule and teach him to complete the activity, put materials away, remove the token or coin from the schedule page, place it on his token board, and then turn the page. When he has filled all of the Velcro dots on his clipboard, guide him to show you (or another adult) the clipboard, and help him exchange his tokens for a special reward.

If your child attempts to "cheat" (takes tokens when he has not completed a scheduled activity or has incorrectly completed it), use the teaching procedures discussed earlier. Remove the token or coin that he did not earn, and guide him to continue his schedule.

As your youngster becomes more proficient, continue to add photographs to the three-ring binder and the choice board, and consider when to move tokens or coins from every page of his schedule book to every second page, and then every third page. Your data on schedule following will be helpful in making this decision.

It is interesting to note that when children gain proficiency at activities that were once quite difficult, the mastered activities often become preferred activities. These previously challenging activities can then be displayed on choice boards and used as rewards. It is the same for all of us. Learning to ride a bicycle, dive off the diving board, or drive a car with a manual gear shift may initially be scary and taxing, but after we learn the relevant skills, we enjoy those endeavors.

Wes

Sixteen-year-old Wes, a member of a large family, follows a photographic schedule that begins when he arrives home from school at three o'clock, and ends at bedtime. His scheduled activities include dusting, vacuuming, making his school lunch for the next day, doing laundry, practicing typing skills, unloading the dishwasher, setting the table, interacting with family members, feeding the dog, doing homework, reporting on completed activities, and occasionally weeding, raking leaves, or shoveling snow.

Initially, each of these tasks was presented in a separate photographic schedule. For example, making a school lunch was, at one time, a sixteen-page schedule that included pictures of a lunch bag, slices of bread, a knife, butter, lunch meat, cheese, a sandwich, a sandwich bag, vegetables, a plastic bag, fruit, a dessert, his initials on the lunch bag, *putting the knife in the dishwasher, wiping the counter with a sponge, and putting the lunch bag in the refrigerator. When Wes learned this separate schedule, it was represented by a single picture in his main photographic schedule (a picture of a bulging lunch bag bearing his initials).*

Over several years, Wes mastered many separate and lengthy schedules, and they are now represented by single photographs in his primary activity schedule, which is more than forty pages in length. He has acquired many leisure skills, and his recreational choices include in-line skating, biking, shooting baskets, kicking a soccer ball, jogging, preparing a variety of foods, swimming, watching TV, playing ping pong with family members, playing video games, and completing puzzles.

Wes selects and sequences all of his daily activities. It is noteworthy that he often chooses to complete all of his work assignments before engaging in leisure activities.

9 | From Pictures to Words

Lee

By age 4, Lee could read a lot of sight words, and we were able to use a number of toys that might not otherwise have been ideal candidates for his picture schedule. For example, we included a picture of a Playskool hammer bench with pegs of six different colors; we arranged the color words in different orders on the page, and taught him to hammer the pegs in the order listed in his schedule. We also used a photograph of Velcro play food that could be "cut" apart, with the words "cut the food," and different word cards listing the foods to be cut. And we cut out a figure of a person, laminated it and clothing of different colors, and displayed a picture of these materials with word cards that told him to "dress the boy," and listed the clothing to use (e.g., blue shirt, white socks). Lee likes singing, so to promote interaction, we put cards in his schedule that said, "Mommy, sing the Alouette song" (and other songs he enjoys).

Introduction

Some children with autism quickly acquire reading skills, but most require a carefully programmed curriculum, such as the Edmark Reading Program (1992). Some youngsters develop early sight-word reading repertoires as a result of incidental teaching procedures (McGee, Krantz, & McClannahan, 1986), and others learn target words that are presented on flash cards during discrete-trial training sessions.

Although many children learn to follow activity schedules before they begin to read, it is important to modify schedule books to recognize these new competencies as they develop. Learning to read enables your child to use a schedule that is more like your own.

Introducing Textual Cues

Sometimes, after a child develops initial reading skills, words can be attached to the photographs in the schedule. Later, the pictures can be removed, with the result that the youngster responds to the words instead of the photographs. On the choice board shown in Figure 9-1, text was superimposed on the pictures. Later, the photographs were removed and only the words remained, and the youngster continued to do the scheduled activities.

But for other young people with autism, more systematic efforts are necessary to prepare them to use written schedules (McClannahan, 1998). Suppose that a youngster especially enjoys bite-size Mounds candy bars, and a picture of a Mounds bar is included in her schedule. The first step in the transition from photograph to text is to replace

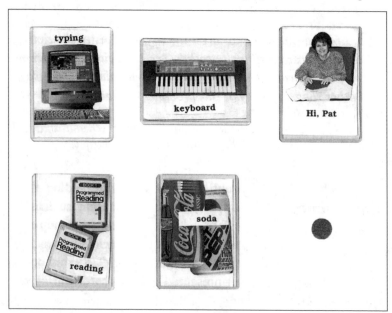

(Fig. 9-1) On this choice board, words are superimposed on photographs.

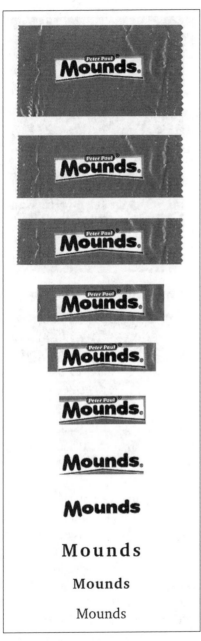

(Fig. 9-2) Steps used to help a child make the transition from a photograph of a Mounds candy bar to the word "Mounds."

the color photo with a black-and-white photo or a photocopy of the candy wrapper. Some next steps are: (a) cut away small sections of the top and bottom of the candy wrapper, (b) cut away the sides of the wrapper, (c) cut away the small words "Peter Paul," and (d) cut away the line under the word (see Figure 9-2). Now only the word "Mounds" remains, but it is presented in special type style. If you have a computer, you may experiment with different type sizes and fonts, to program a gradual transition to a typical type size and style. If you are not a computer user, you can achieve the same outcome by printing the word a little smaller on each presentation. Of course, each next step should be taken only if the child makes a correct response. If she is prompted, or obtains materials other than the Mounds bar, it is important to return to the previous step and provide practice opportunities.

The procedure described in the preceding paragraph is called stimulus fading. When designing stimulus-fading programs, it is important to identify stimuli that are and are not criterion related. Criterion-related stimuli are never faded; they are the stimuli that have

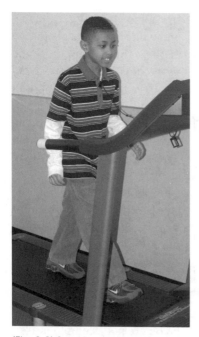

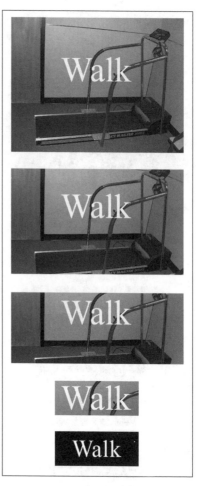

(Fig. 9-3) Superimposition and background fading used to teach sight-word reading.
(above) EJ learned to read 15 new sight words in 24 school days while doing physical education activities.
(right) Words such as "walk" were superimposed on digital photographs and then the backgrounds were faded.

an impact on your behavior, and they have an effect on the behavior of most people in our society. In our example, color and size are not criterion related because they will not help the child read the word "Mounds" when it appears on her choice board or on a flash card in a typical type size and type style. The word "Mounds" is criterion related. When they are well-designed, stimulus-fading programs result in fewer errors and faster learning (Etzel & LeBlanc, 1979).

If pictures in activity schedules do not include words, then words may be superimposed on pictures to help young people make the transition to written schedules. For example, six-year-old EJ learned to follow several different photographic activity schedules, but his progress in reading was slow. His teacher used his gym activity schedule and superimposition and background fading procedures to help him learn to use a written activity schedule (Birkan, McClannahan, and Krantz, 2007). EJ's picture schedule for gym contained fifteen digital photographs of exercise equipment such as jogging trampoline, balance beam, and treadmill. Using a computer program (Adobe Photo Shop) words were superimposed on the center of each photograph. For example, the word "tramp" appeared on the picture of the trampoline, and "walk" was superimposed on the photo of the treadmill.

EJ's instructor used the familiar procedures to teach him to follow his gym schedule, with the exception that if he did not label a depicted activity (or later, read a sight word), the teacher modeled the word while manually guiding him to point to the text. After EJ learned to label each picture in his schedule, background fading began. Fading occurred in five phases. In the first and second phases, 1-centimeter strips were cut and removed from the top and bottom of each photograph; in the third phase, the pictures were cut to show only the text and small portions of the color photographs that showed through the words. In the next phase (needed for only five words), Adobe Photo Shop was used to remove background color from the portions of the photographs that remained visible. And in the final phase, only the words remained on the pages of the activity schedule.

In five months, EJ learned only 16 sight words in his classroom reading program, but with superimposition and background fading procedures, he learned 15 sight words in 24 days. The teaching strategy was time-efficient, because EJ learned to read the words while at the same time completing physical education activities. But most importantly, he began a transition from photographic to written activity schedules.

Although stimulus fading procedures are often helpful in achieving a transition from pictures to text, other strategies have also been shown to be effective. In one investigation (McGee et. al., 1986), two children with autism acquired functional reading skills in the context of an incidental teaching activity. When a child gestured toward or requested a toy, he or she was allowed to play with it after selecting a corresponding word. The results showed that, after teaching, the children read the target words with comprehension, and they read them when they were presented in a different size and type style, and when they were presented in a book rather than on index cards.

Fig. 9-4 | To-Do List Example
To-do lists that cue household tasks, food preparation, and self-care. The youngster places a check mark to the left of each item after completing it.

Clean the Sink

____ Get bucket from broom closet

____ Put gloves on

____ Take things off sink

____ Spray mirror with Windex

____ Wipe mirror with paper towel

____ Look for streaks

____ Spray sink with Windex

____ Wipe with paper towel

____ Look for dirt

____ Put things back on sink

____ Put Windex and towels in bucket

____ Take off gloves

____ Put gloves in bucket

____ Put bucket in broom closet

____ Wash hands

____ Ask Mom, "How does the sink look?"

Make Pudding

____ Wash hands

____ Get bowl

____ Get measuring cup

____ Get milk

____ Fill cup with milk

____ Pour milk in dish

____ Put measuring cup in dishwasher

____ Put milk away

____ Get box of pudding

____ Get scissors

___ Open box
___ Cut bag open
___ Put pudding mix in bowl
___ Throw box away
___ Put scissors away
___ Get whisk
___ Set timer for 2 minutes
___ Stir pudding
___ Turn timer off
___ Put lid on bowl
___ Put bowl in refrigerator
___ Set timer for 5 minutes
___ Put whisk in dishwasher
___ Wipe counter
___ Get 2 little bowls
___ Get 2 napkins
___ Get one big spoon
___ Ask Jimmy, "Do you want pudding?"

Shave
___ Get shaving kit
___ Turn razor on
___ Shave left cheek
___ Shave right cheek
___ Shave under nose
___ Shave chin
___ Shave neck
___ Turn razor off
___ Check for whiskers
___ Clean razor
___ Put razor in shaving kit
___ Put shaving kit away
___ Clean sink

Other researchers (Miguel, Yang, Finn and Ahern, 2009) used a match-to-sample procedure to help children move from pictures to printed words in their schedules. The children were taught to select pictures and printed words that matched the words dictated by an experimenter. After training, the two preschoolers with autism "could respond to printed words by completing the depicted task, match printed words to pictures, and read printed words without explicit training. . . ." (p. 703).

Reading Skills and "To-Do" Lists

Reading skills create many new opportunities for independence and choice, because activities are more efficiently represented by words than by photographs. When a child begins to use textual rather than photographic cues, you may, at least for a while, continue the familiar format. Allow him to select word cards from his choice board and notebook and place them in his schedule book. But when he is following his schedule with minimal errors, it is time to introduce the "to-do" list.

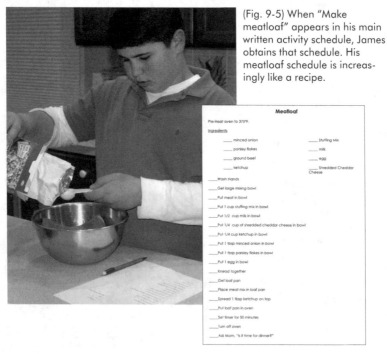

(Fig. 9-5) When "Make meatloaf" appears in his main written activity schedule, James obtains that schedule. His meatloaf schedule is increasingly like a recipe.

Meatloaf

Pre-Heat oven to 375°F.

Ingredients

____ minced onion	____ Stuffing Mix
____ parsley flakes	____ milk
____ ground beef	____ egg
____ ketchup	____ Shredded Cheddar Cheese

____Wash Hands

____Get large mixing bowl

____Put meat in bowl

____Put 1 cup stuffing mix in bowl

____Put 1/2 cup milk in bowl

____Put 1/4 cup of shredded cheddar cheese in bowl

____Put 1/4 cup ketchup in bowl

____Put 1 tbsp minced onion in bowl

____Put 1 tbsp parsley flakes in bowl

____Put 1 egg in bowl

____Knead together

____Get loaf pan

____Place meat mix in loaf pan

____Spread 1 tbsp ketchup on top

____Put loaf pan in oven

____Set timer for 50 minutes

____Turn off oven

____Ask Mom, "Is it time for dinner?"

Using words that are mastered, sequence them in a list that will guide the child through a series of responses. To-do lists may be used to cue household chores, food preparation, or self-care activities, as well as homework, exercise, and social interaction tasks.

If a youngster has paper-and-pencil skills, place a blank to the left of each item on the list, and teach him to check off each activity after it is accomplished (see Figure 9-4). If pencil use is a problem, put a Velcro dot to the left of each item, and teach him to move a coin or token to the next task in the list (see Figure 9-6). Teach to-do lists in the same way that you taught your child to use his first schedules. When you present the list for the first time, be prepared to use manual guidance, and the familiar prompting and prompt-fading procedures.

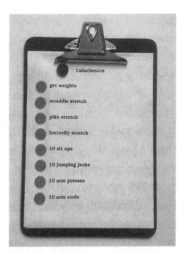

(Fig. 9-6) A to-do list for a workout. After completing each task, the youth moves the coin to the next task.

Learning to use a to-do list is a key accomplishment! Many adults also use to-do lists to remind them of exercises during workouts, Saturday errands, grocery purchases, and phone calls.

Using Appointment Books

As reading and handwriting skills progress, some young people begin to use appointment books that are much like our own. Words that were previously presented on the choice board or in a notebook are transferred to 3 x 5 note cards that are placed in a file box. Using the familiar instructional procedures, we manually guide the individual to remove the cards from the box, lay them on a work surface, sequence the activity cards, and record them in an appointment book in the order he selected. After the schedule is constructed, we use manual guidance and prompt-fading to teach him to check off or cross out each activity after it is completed (see Figure 1-3, page 6). We know some young people who spend thirty minutes or more each day arranging note cards and constructing their own schedules. We do not view this as a problem, but as an indication that they care about their schedules.

Selection of an appointment book or daily planner may be determined by the size of a young person's handwriting. If his writing is large, provide a desk-size planner and gradually diminish the space between lines. If his handwriting permits, buy a smaller appointment book.

For many young people, appointment books or planners are their main schedules; these primary schedules refer the users to many sub-schedules. At age 10, Thomas has many sub-schedules. For example, when the main schedule in his daily planner refers him to math, he obtains the notebook that contains his arithmetic assignment and the relevant worksheets, takes the materials to his desk, and completes the assignment. Then he raises his hand and asks the teacher to check his work. After he and the teacher review his answers, he puts the materials away, returns to his daily planner, and checks off the activity to show that it was completed.

On some days, his schedule includes food preparation. He obtains the notebook that contains the recipes that he has previously mastered and the to-do list that he is using to learn to prepare a new food—chicken noodle casserole. Some tasks that were in his previous food-preparation schedules are no longer included in his new recipes because he has acquired those skills. For example, he no longer needs separate written cues to wash his hands, open cans, or put dirty dishes and utensils in the dishwasher. Some of his other sub-schedules include reading, spelling, typing, tooth brushing, gym, and talking to peers during lunch.

Activity Schedules in a High-Tech World

Today, youngsters who grow up with activity schedules may learn to use schedules that are presented on desktop or hand-held computers. Schedules on desk-top computers may be best for young children who are acquiring early schedule-following skills and who are not yet ready for activities that require moving from room to room. PowerPoint software can be used to create desk-top computer schedules that include photos, sounds, text, and videos (Rehfeldt, Kinney, Root, & Stromer, 2004).

Older children, teens, and adults with autism who have learned to follow photographic or written schedules may next learn to use schedules presented on personal digital assistants (PDAs), also referred to as

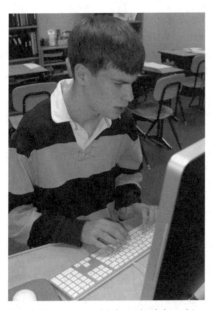

(Fig. 9-7) Tommy adds his schedule to his pocket computer.

hand-held or pocket computers. Hand-held computers such as the Apple iPod touch, Archos, and Microsoft Zune can present digital photographs, text, or both. In our settings, children as young as nine learn to use photographic or written schedules that appear on hand-held devices; they use the stylus or touch screen to check off each activity when it is completed. Initially, youngsters may use a stylus or touch screen too vigorously, or may not take care to avoid damaging digital devices, but manual guidance and prompt fading (and sometimes, token loss) usually solve these problems. Many users may not yet have learned to add their own schedules to their PDAs, so teachers or parents perform this task for them. Later, older children, teens, and adults with autism are taught to add their own schedules to their hand-held devices; of course, they complete this task using written or photographic activity schedules. (See Figure 9-7.)

Recently, one group of researchers (Mechling, Gast, and Seid, 2009) used a personal digital assistant (PDA) with photographic, auditory, and video prompts with voice-over to teach students with autism spectrum disorder to prepare Hamburger Helper and toaster-oven pizza. These researchers reported that the adolescents' skills in completing the recipes maintained over time. However, it may be important to note that multiple cues (for example, photographs *and* video *and* sounds *and* voice-over) may delay young people's development of independence because ultimately, many of these prompts should be faded.

Today, pocket computers are ubiquitous, and their widespread use is advantageous to young people with autism. Activity schedules in notebooks can be cumbersome and may draw attention in community settings, but activity schedules on PDAs are less visible. However, pocket computers are expensive. In addition, researchers who compared the use of a photographic schedule presented in a three-ring binder versus a photographic schedule presented on a PDA found no difference in performance; both formats were associated with sustained engagement and high task completion (Decker, Ferrigno, May, Natoli, Olson, Schaefer, Cammilleri, and Brothers, 2003).

10 | Expanding Social Interaction Skills

Introduction

Chapter 3 describes how to include social activities in children's first activity schedules. This chapter explains how to program more complex social interaction tasks. Of course, these endeavors will be most successful if you begin at your child's current language level.

Social Skills for Nonverbal Children

Youngsters who have not yet acquired speech can learn to initiate social activities. For example, you may teach a child to remove a picture of a swing, wagon, or bubbles from her schedule book, choice board, or notebook and give it to you as a means of beginning a social activity with you. Although she cannot yet talk, she can learn to seek you out, get your attention, and begin a social exchange, so that you can model conversation.

Later you may display photographs of family members or therapists on her choice board and teach her to select both the activity and the person with whom she will do it. Guide her to choose a photograph of an activity, select a photograph of a person, attach the picture of the person to the card on which the activity photo is mounted, and, finally, seek out that family member and hand the card to him or her, as a means of beginning a social activity.

Offer social activities that your child enjoys. Depending on her preferences, you may read (or label pictures in) a favorite book, play with musical or noise-making toys, make block towers for her to knock over, play games with a flashlight, help her ride a trike, or jog her on your knees. If her visual attending skills are not yet well developed, you can build them by waiting for her to look at you before you accept the card and begin the activity she selected.

Children with autism often fail to "recruit attention" from others—that is, they don't point to or show objects to others for the purpose of sharing a social experience. For example, they don't show parents pictures they colored, point out objects of interest, or ask parents to watch them engage in play activities. They may also engage in stereotypic or disruptive behavior that parents inadvertently reinforce by attending to it. If this pattern continues over time, children's disruptive behavior becomes more frequent and they fall farther behind their peers in developing skills that gain attention for appropriate behavior. There is a message here: Start early and continue to teach social initiations as your child develops additional language.

Kirk

On the ride home from school, six-year-old Kirk often cried and kicked the back of the car seat if his mother selected a different route or stopped to run an errand. His mother took a proactive approach—she took pictures of all of the places they might stop and put them in an album, one photo per page. A button-activated voice recorder, attached with Velcro to the front of the album, played the recorded question, "Where are we going?" The last page in the album was a photograph of their house. A token was attached to the bottom of each page of the album, and there were Velcro dots on the album cover.

Before each ride, Kirk's mother removed, re-sequenced, or replaced pictures in the album, depending on the day's agenda. After completing an errand, such as leaving the drive-through window at the bank, she said, "We're finished at the bank—give yourself a token" or "We're done with banking; you earned a token." If Kirk kicked or cried, he did not earn tokens and if he gave himself an unearned token, his mother pulled into a safe parking area, stopped the car, and removed his album and tokens. But when Kirk earned all of his tokens, he chose a special reward upon his arrival home.

During the first practice trips, Kirk's teenage sister (who had been briefed by her mother) rode along to guide him through his car-ride schedule. After a few practice rides, Kirk eagerly got in the car and checked his schedule; disruptive behavior was now minimal or absent. Two weeks later, upon entering the car, Kirk asked, "Where are we going?" without using the button-activated recorder. After he did this on three consecutive rides, the recorder was removed and he continued to initiate conversation with his mother about stops on the way home.

Social Skills for Children Who Say a Few Words

If you have other children, you know that typical preschoolers often say such things as, "Look," "Watch me," "What's that?" "Where's Daddy?" and "All done." These verbal productions can be included in youngsters' activity schedules, using a card reader or button-activated voice recorder. This enables the child to initiate the interaction, and helps to diminish the likelihood that he will become dependent on verbal prompts from you.

After recording models of the words you want a child to imitate, put the recordings in the activity schedule in the order that they will be used. If you are using a card reader and cards, the cards can be attached with Velcro if you place the Velcro buttons at the top of the cards, above the portion that runs through the card reader. If you are using a relatively flat button-activated voice recorder such as the Voice-Over (see Appendix C), attach the voice recorders to pages of the activity schedule.

If you record the word "Look," arrange the schedule book so that the card or button-activated recorder with the recorded word follows an activity in which your child creates a product he can show you. For example, after he completes a coloring task, puzzle, or bristle block tower, guide him to bring the finished product to you or another family member, remove the card or button-activated recorder from the schedule, play the recorded word, and say, "Look." If you record the words "Watch me," place the photo of the card or button-activated voice recorder before a depicted activity for which you can be the audience. Teach your child to play the recorded script, imitate "Watch me," and then do a somersault, jump on a jogging trampoline, throw a ball, or run a truck down the ramp.

When he says "Look" or "Watch me," respond enthusiastically, but don't ask him for more language (this isn't a discrete-trial teaching session). Instead, make statements that he can understand, and that you hope will be of interest to him (e.g., "You colored ice cream!" or "Barney puzzle!" or "Red fire truck!"). Then look expectantly at him, and wait to see if he has anything else to say. (If he doesn't, you can make another simple statement, such as "Barney is purple.") Research shows that over a period of time, he may combine your words with words he already knows, to produce new statements such as "Look, Barney" or "Big fire truck" (Krantz & McClannahan, 1998).

Initially, when you add these social activities to the activity schedule, it's important to arrange the environment to promote success. Put the activity schedule and card reader near the toy shelf. Sit on the floor or on a small chair so that you are at the youngster's eye level, and sit near the schedule so that you can prompt quickly to prevent errors.

Use the familiar manual guidance and prompt-fading procedures to teach your child to use the card reader or button-activated recorder, approach and orient toward you, imitate the recorded words, and display a product or show you an activity. If he plays but doesn't imitate a recording, manually guide him to play it again (and again), but don't use verbal prompts. If you find that he is unable to imitate recorded words, consider providing discrete-trial training to imitate recorded words before putting them back in his schedule.

When your child masters these first social tasks, add more. A recorded script such as "Where's Daddy?" may be an opportunity to take a walk around the house to find a parent who will provide a tickle or a toss in the air. And the script "Where's doggy?" may set the occasion to take a brief walk in the yard and play with the family pet.

When your child becomes more proficient in playing a recorded script, approaching and orienting toward you, and saying the script, you may decide to move farther away from the activity schedule, so that the youngster learns to seek out conversation partners. These procedures are described in detail in *Teaching Conversation to Children with Autism: Scripts and Script Fading* (McClannahan and Krantz, 2005).

Building Peer Interaction Skills

Learning to observe and imitate the behavior of others is important to the development of social interaction skills. Parents often model words or phrases for their babies—for example, "Bye bye," "Mmm good," "All gone," "Dada," and "Mama"—and typical infants soon begin to imitate these models. But many children with autism need special instruction to learn to imitate, and even after they dependably imitate models provided by teachers and parents, they may not imitate the responses of other children. Teaching peer imitation is a first step in the development of peer interaction repertoires.

In our settings, beginning peer imitation programs are carefully structured. Two children sit at a table, facing one another. Each child has an identical set of three toys on the table in front of him or her, and an adult sits or stands behind each youngster. One child has an activity schedule that contains pictures of each toy. One adult guides the child to open the schedule book and point to and use the depicted toy. The other adult guides the second child to imitate the play behavior of her peer. Both children receive tokens—one for modeling the depicted play activity, and the other for imitating the model. When the activity schedule is completed, both children exchange their tokens for a special reward and then the peer "teacher" and "student" exchange roles.

Prompts for "teacher" and "student" are faded in the usual fashion, beginning with graduated guidance. When both children follow the activity schedule and imitate one another when the adults' proximity is faded to one or two feet, photographs in the schedule are re-sequenced and toys are placed on the table in a different order.

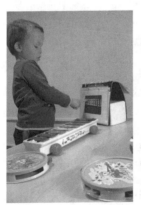 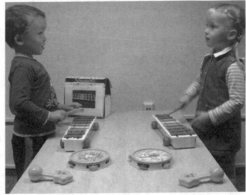

(Fig. 10-1) *(left)* In Gdansk, Poland, Jacek plays the role of teacher; he points to a picture in his activity schedule.
(right) When he models behavior such as playing the xylophone, his twin, Aleksandra, imitates. Later, Aleksandra will be the peer tutor and it will be Jacek's turn to imitate the responses she models.

After a child reliably imitates the play behavior of a peer model, it is important to teach her to imitate other responses, such as waving, jumping, clapping, or sitting down. If a youngster has learned to say the alphabet, the activity schedule may cue her to instruct her peer, "Get A," and the second child responds by finding the target letter and putting it in the alphabet puzzle. Other activity schedules may cue the young "teacher" to instruct her peer to "Find 2," or "Get cow." Of course, the goal is to move beyond this highly structured format and to teach cooperative play activities, such as jointly doing puzzles; following one another down the slide; chasing one another on the playground; running races; playing games (Betz, Higbee, and Reagon, 2008); or initiating interaction while playing with toys (Wichnick, Vener, Keating, and Poulson, 2010).

Social Skills for Children Who Use Phrases and Sentences

Adults often speak about things they have done and things they are going to do. Recorded scripts or written scripts (if your child reads) can help youngsters with autism do the same. For example, a child's activity schedule may cue her to report, "I'm going to cut," or "I finished handwriting." Data from the Princeton Child Development Institute's preschool and school suggest that, for children with sufficient language, providing several examples of a communication may help to expand language use. For example, the child who is about to use scissors and paste may select from one of three scripts: "I'm going to cut," "It's time to paste," and "I like to cut." And when cutting and pasting is completed, she may again select from three different communications, such as "Cutting is fun," "I finished cutting," and "Pasting is over."

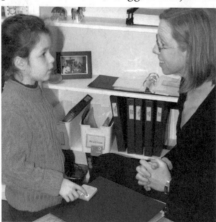

(Fig. 10-2) Martha presses a button to play the partially faded script, "Writing..." and tells her teacher, "Writing is fun." The teacher replies, "You wrote Mom!"

Textual and auditory scripts help youngsters learn to give and receive information about themselves and others, and to enlist others' participation in activities. For example, a young child may imitate a recorded model by saying "Let's go," or "Come with me" while taking the hand of a classmate or sibling and moving toward a depicted wagon or seesaw. Scripts such as "What are you doing?" or "What's this?" typically produce responses, not only from parents, but also from siblings, peers, and relatives. And young people with more speech or reading skills many initiate conversation with statements or questions such as "I like Burger King," "What's your favorite restaurant?" "Tony is my friend," "Do you have a pet?" or "Do you like music?"

Remember that these initiations should not be met with a barrage of questions, but with statements that the child is likely to understand and that are of interest to her. Social interaction skills are difficult for children with autism and they are more likely to learn that interaction is rewarding if we don't respond with difficult questions or demands for more language. Figure 10-3 shows a conversation between Ron, age 9, and his teacher. Ron enjoys camping with his family, and some of his previous recorded scripts have addressed this topic. Note that

---

Fig. 10-3 | A Recorded Script

This conversation between Ron and his teacher was initiated by Ron, after he played a recorded script. Note that the teacher does not ask questions or give directions, but makes statements that are of interest to Ron.

Ron: (Says recorded script). I go camping with Mom and Dad.
Teacher: You have a sleeping bag.
Ron: I sleep tent.
Teacher: You camp by the river.
Ron: By the river . . . I swim.
Teacher: You're a good swimmer! (Then broadens topic to promote Ron's response.) And you ride in the boat.
Ron: Boat . . . I like boats.
Teacher: I like boats, too. And I like to cook hot dogs when I camp.
Ron: I like hot dogs.
Teacher: I put mustard and catsup on my hot dogs.
Ron: (No response after ten seconds)
Teacher: It's nice talking to you.
Ron: Nice talking to you. (Returns to schedule).

the teacher does not ask questions or give directions, but guides the conversation in ways that encourage Ron's participation.

Fading Auditory and Textual Cues

After your child learns to use recorded scripts or written words to initiate social interaction, help him take the next steps toward independence by gradually eliminating these cues. For example, if the recorded script was "What are you doing?" and he always says this script, begin by deleting the last word, so that the recording now plays the words "What are you." If your child continues to say the entire script on two or three occasions, delete another word, so that the recorder now plays "What are." If he makes an error, return to the prior step ("What are you"), but if he correctly says the script on several opportunities, fade to "What." Eventually erase "What" and provide a blank card or a button-activated recorder without a message (Stevenson, Krantz, and McClannahan, 1998).

When encountering a blank card or voice recorder, many youngsters behave as though the card reader or button-activated recorder is broken—they push the buttons and play the card several times before they say the script. If your child does not say the script when it is absent, use manual guidance to help him put the card or button-activated recorder away and turn toward you. If he still does not say the script, return to the previous step (a recording that plays "What"). Finally, when your child says the script when it is absent, add a new script and begin the process again, in order to teach him more conversation skills.

Script-fading procedures are similar for young readers. If a girl consistently reads the words "Do you like to sing?" the text is faded to "Do you like to," and if she continues to respond correctly, the script is faded to "Do you like" and so on, until only a generic cue (such as the word "Talk") remains in her activity schedule (Krantz & McClannahan, 1993).

Marcus

Marcus, age 7, appeared to enjoy playing the piano but never talked about it. Because he had some reading skills, his teacher created scripts about his piano playing. Scripts such as "I'm going to practice piano,"

"Listen to this," and "That was my favorite song" were written on index cards. Next, his teacher asked him to read the target sentences, and if he did not read some words, or read them incorrectly, she put those words on flash cards and taught him to read them before the scripts were added to his activity schedule. Scripts appeared in Marcus's written schedule before and after daily piano practice and after he dependably read them, they were gradually faded from last word to first word. For example, the script "I'm going to practice piano" was faded to "I'm going to practice," then "I'm going to," then "I'm going," then "I'm," and then the script was absent and only a blank card appeared in his schedule.

After several sets of scripts were introduced and faded, Marcus turned a page of his daily activity schedule and found the piano schedule shown in Figure 10-4. His teacher guided him to point to the word "Talk" in his schedule, prominently displayed one of his tokens, and waited. After a few seconds, Marcus said, "I'm going to practice piano."

Figure 10-4 shows Marcus's piano schedule, as well as Marcus interacting with his teacher.

Practice Piano

___ **Talk**

___ **Play Song 1**

___ **Talk**

___ **Play Song 2**

___ **Talk**

___ **Play Song 3**

___ **Talk**

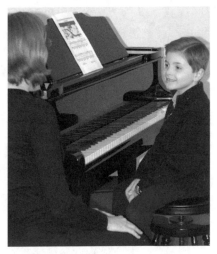

(Fig. 10-4) *(above left)* Marcus's piano schedule helps him interact with listeners.

(right) After playing the first piece, he turns to his teacher and says, "I played Yankee Doodle."

11 | Activity Schedules for Adults

Some young people with autism who received intervention at the Princeton Child Development Institute (PCDI) made successful transitions to public schools and are now adults who are indistinguishable from the rest of us. Their educational achievements and careers are quite varied, but they use the same prompt systems and reminders that we use. Of the teenagers and adults who continue to receive services at PCDI, some have been schedule followers since they were toddlers. But this technology is relatively recent, and others did not learn to use schedules until they were adults. It is never too late to teach a person with autism to follow an activity schedule.

But in the best of circumstances, preparation for adulthood begins long before learners arrive at age twenty-one. We must begin early to help children acquire skills that will be called for in adulthood (Mc-Clannahan, MacDuff, & Krantz, 2002). These skill sets include:

- accepting manual guidance,
- following pictorial or written activity schedules,
- requesting assistance when relevant,
- making choices and sequencing one's own activities,
- initiating social interaction,
- completing tasks without continuous supervision,
- delivering one's own rewards, and
- completing activities of long duration that include many separate responses.

Beyond childhood, activity schedules continue to help adults develop critical repertoires. They help them learn to complete ever longer and more elaborate response sequences; to complete home-living tasks and interact with other members of their households; to develop skills that are essential to employment; and to participate in community life.

Activity Schedules at Home

Of the older adolescents and adults enrolled in PCDI's programs, some live at home with their parents, some live in group homes, and others make their homes in supervised apartments. Regardless of the type of home environment, home living requires a plethora of skills. The following paragraphs describe how activity schedules enabled three young people with autism—Patrick, Tony, and Kate—to gain skills that maximize their independence.

Patrick

Patrick lives at home with his parents and two younger siblings. He is not a reader. His main photographic schedule directs him to many sub-schedules, and many steps in his activities are now represented by single visual cues (Mechling, Gast, & Seid, 2009). His shaving schedule, for example, previously consisted of eighteen pictures, but shaving is now represented by a single photograph; the same is true of taking a shower, clipping nails, and applying acne cream—all of these were once separate schedules.

Patrick has not learned to select clothing that is appropriate to the season, nor does he select matching or complementary colors. For this reason, his parents took photographs of shirts and pants that "go together" and placed them in a choice book. Each morning, he selects one of the pictures, places it in his schedule, finds the depicted items of clothing, and independently gets dressed.

Some time ago, Patrick learned to follow schedules to wash and dry clothes; subsequently, a single picture of the washer and dryer cued him to help with the laundry. However, his mother continued to sort the laundry, because Patrick had difficulty sorting clothing into light and dark loads. But she solved the problem using a color printer. She printed gradations of light colors and gradations of dark colors and taped a color gradient to each of two laundry baskets. *A picture of the two laundry baskets full of light- and dark-colored clothing was placed in Patrick's schedule, and his mother used manual guidance and prompt-fading procedures to help him match items of clothing to the sample colors taped to the laundry baskets and sort them into different baskets.*

Other home living tasks that were taught with photographic activity schedules include setting the table, loading and unloading the dishwasher, cleaning his room, and preparing food. Patrick has learned to make toast, scrambled eggs, and oatmeal for breakfast; several different types of sandwiches and salads for lunch; and dinners that include spaghetti and meatballs, shepherd's pie, and tuna casserole.

Although Patrick can speak, he does not often initiate conversation, so his activity schedule includes social interaction tasks. Photographs of numbered, button-activated voice recorders are placed in his main activity schedule, and matching numerals appear on the recorders that are kept on a shelf near his sub-schedules. When he turns to a page that displays a voice recorder, he obtains the matching recorder and finds an available family member. Sample scripts are, "What are you doing?" "Is there anything I can do to help?" "I'm going to ____," and "I finished ____." Patrick usually completes open-ended sentences without help. Other scripts help him initiate activities with his siblings (for example, "Do you want to play dominoes?").

A photograph of a choice book in Patrick's main schedule cues leisure activities. The choice book contains pictures of video games, MP3 player, puzzles, in-line skates, computer, snacks, television, and bike. Patrick has learned to set a kitchen timer, and numbers attached to the pictures indicate the number of minutes allotted to each activity. When necessary, his parents adjust these times to help him coordinate his activities with those of other family members.

Although graduated guidance and prompt fading procedures are needed when Patrick is learning new skills, his activity schedules enable him to be quite independent at home, and he makes many contributions to his household.

Tony

Tony lived in a group home during adolescence, but now shares an apartment with another young adult with autism. As a teenager, he used a photographic schedule, but now uses textual cues. Reading did not come

*easily for him, and he continues to learn new sight words before they are
added to his written schedules.*

*Like his roommate, Tony uses daily, weekly, and monthly schedules.
His daily schedule includes activities similar to those of most adults.
Portions of his weekly and monthly schedules are shown in Figure 11-1.*

Fig. 11-1 | Sample Weekly and Monthly Schedules for Tony

Date	Weekly Activities
5/23/09	Clean refrigerator
5/23/09	Clean kitchen
	Clean bathroom
5/18/09	Plan menus
5/19/09	Inventory groceries
5/19/09	Inventory drug store supplies
5/19/09	Make shopping list
	Schedule shopping trip. Shop on ____
5/20/09	Plan an outing. Go to **movie** on 5/24/09
	Vacuum and dust
5/18, 20, 22/09	Make dinner (Mondays, Wednesdays, and Fridays)
	Strip bed and do laundry
5/18/09	Weigh and write weight (Monday). Weight is 195
	Manage mail
5/17, 19, 21/09	Ride exercise bike (3 times a week)
Date	**Monthly Activities**
5/18/09	Make haircut appointment
	Wash jackets
	Clean oven
5/23/09	Pay cell phone bill by the 25th (due the 1st)
	Pay rent by the 5th (due the 10th)
	Pay phone bill by the 7th (due the 12th)
	Pay cable bill by the 10th (due the 15th)

When Tony plans dinner menus, he refers to his "cookbook," which contains all of the recipes (written activity schedules) for tasks he previously mastered, as well as those for foods he is currently learning to prepare. Tony selects some recipes that he will prepare in the coming week, and writes the necessary ingredients on his shopping list. He has lists of all of the drugstore supplies that he regularly uses (such as toothpaste, deodorant, and shave cream), as well as kitchen staples. When he inventories his grocery and drug store supplies, he uses these lists and crosses off items that are present; the remaining items are transferred to his shopping list. These skills were taught with activity schedules.

Tony regularly washes his jackets because his job involves outdoor ground maintenance, such as picking up trash on lawns. Paying bills is difficult for him because reading and handwriting are not preferred activities. For that reason, he pays one bill at a time, but nevertheless pays his bills on time. His schedules of meal preparation and housekeeping tasks ensure that he and his roommate have an equitable division of home-living responsibilities.

Tony also has an activity schedule that helps him entertain guests. Initially, his schedule included items relevant to inviting guests; planning and preparing snacks or meals; receiving guests (including checking to make certain that a person at the door is a familiar person, not a stranger); serving food; initiating and continuing conversation; and leave taking. Now, this schedule is a short list of reminders.

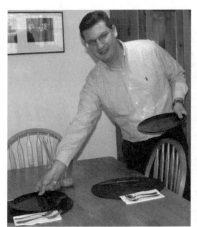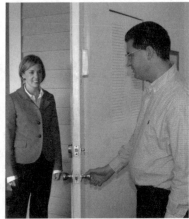

(Fig. 11-2) *(left)* On his day off, Tony sets the table and prepares to receive a guest for lunch. *(right)* He greets his visitor and invites her into his apartment.

Kate

Kate, age 27, uses the iCal program on her Mac computer to keep track of weekly, monthly, and yearly tasks and events (the equivalent program for PCs is Outlook). A written activity schedule helped her learn to use iCal, and her daily schedule reminds her to refer to her calendar on the computer screen or to print a hard copy. Annual reminders on her calendar indicate when she should schedule physical, dental, and eye exams. After appointments are made, she enters those dates and times on the calendar. Family members' birthdays are calendar entries that prompt her to send greeting cards or purchase gifts. Social invitations from peers, visits to her parents' home, and other special occasions also appear on her calendar. In addition, items on her calendar often suggest topics of conversation. Kate appears to enjoy discussing her next visits with family members, her plans for the next holiday, or her Christmas gift list.

As an adolescent, Kate used a written activity schedule to learn to use e-mail (See Figure 11-3). A companion schedule helped her learn to write brief communications: items on that schedule cued her to write a greeting, write an opening comment or question, provide information about one or more of her activities, make a closing comment, and end with her name. Now Kate no longer needs detailed schedules to help her communicate with friends and family—an entry in her main schedule cues her to e-mail. She carries on correspondence with her aunts and uncles, with her siblings who are away at college, and with peers. Activity schedules launched opportunities for interaction that will continue throughout her life.

Activity Schedules at Work

Motivational Systems

Preparing young people for the world of work means, among other things, teaching them to value money. Token systems that feature coins and bills can help to achieve this objective. We look forward to our paychecks because they enable us to purchase valued items, such as groceries, housing, clothing, and vacations. Similarly, coins attached to a clipboard acquire value for young people with autism because the coins are exchanged for preferred foods and activities. And after people

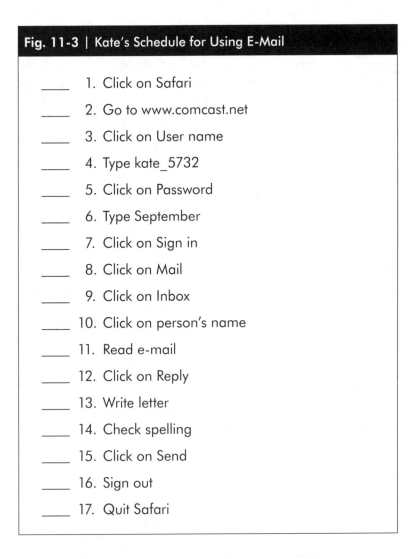

Fig. 11-3 | Kate's Schedule for Using E-Mail

____ 1. Click on Safari

____ 2. Go to www.comcast.net

____ 3. Click on User name

____ 4. Type kate_5732

____ 5. Click on Password

____ 6. Type September

____ 7. Click on Sign in

____ 8. Click on Mail

____ 9. Click on Inbox

____ 10. Click on person's name

____ 11. Read e-mail

____ 12. Click on Reply

____ 13. Write letter

____ 14. Check spelling

____ 15. Click on Send

____ 16. Sign out

____ 17. Quit Safari

learn to count coins, they may exchange them for dollars that are later used to purchase other rewards that they value. These procedures are helpful, not only because they teach people to value money and want to earn it, but also because they help them learn to remain engaged when reinforcement is delayed.

In most employment situations, monetary rewards (paychecks) are delivered only after weeks of work, but most adults with autism need intermediate rewards that help to bridge the delay. These rewards should be as inconspicuous as possible. Although some people may continue to need tokens that are coins, these may be placed on pages of a photographic schedule and moved to the inside cover of the notebook after each depicted task is completed. Of course, if a young person gives himself a coin when he did not complete a task, or incorrectly completed it, a parent, instructor, or job coach must remove the token.

Some adults with autism carry a certain number of coins in a left pocket and move one coin from the left to the right pocket after completing each task. When all coins have been transferred to the right pocket, the person exchanges them for a reward. Other people use wrist counters like those worn by golfers; the counter is advanced each time a task is completed, and points are exchanged for rewards when the counter shows a specified number. Still other workers may tally numbers on an index card that is kept in a pocket and exchange these "points" for a reward after arriving at a designated total.

These strategies help people tolerate longer delays before receiving rewards, and enable them to use less-conspicuous reinforcement systems that do not detract from their competence in community workplaces.

Choices at Work

Young workers with autism, like us, should have opportunities to make choices about their job placements and their daily work agendas; activity schedules are helpful in this regard (McClannahan, MacDuff, and Krantz, 2002).

Julio

As a teenager, Julio learned to use written schedules that cued him to do word processing and data entry tasks, file documents, weed and mulch flower beds, and sweep patios and sidewalks. Later, he was given choices about which tasks to complete. Although his keyboard skills were excellent and he seldom made errors when filing, he consistently chose outdoor tasks that involved manual labor, even when those tasks required a greater time commitment than computer work. Although Julio didn't have sufficient communication skills to express his employment interests, his choices of tasks made his job preferences quite clear. For several years, he has been employed by a local organic farm and he says that he likes his job.

Harry

Harry, who is employed as a hotel housekeeper, uses a photographic activity schedule. Pictures of the many tasks associated with cleaning a hotel room were loaded onto his iPod touch, using the photo album feature. Harry's job coach learned how to do the job himself before he took the photographs and put them on the pocket computer; then he used manual guidance and prompt fading to teach the relevant housekeeping skills. Because Harry was an experienced schedule follower, he quickly achieved criterion performances on the new tasks. After he cleans a room, he looks at each photo again—this time to check his work, and then he moves the last coin from his left pocket to his right pocket. Then he chooses a video game on his hand-held computer and briefly plays it before going to clean the next room. Many contemporary pocket computers accommodate multiple photographic activity schedules as well as multiple leisure-time applications.

Work Schedules and Break Time

Chris uses a pocket computer to view his written schedule; he easily navigates from his main schedule to his sub-schedules. He also uses an application that serves as a digital check register, and he is learning to use the clock feature to program multiple alarms that will remind him to keep appointments or take breaks.

For many employees with autism, taking a break is a repertoire that must be taught. Although they may be excellent schedule followers, sitting quietly in a cafeteria or lunch room or talking with co-workers can be challenging. Photographic or written activity schedules address these skill deficits. For example, George's conversational skills were limited, so he

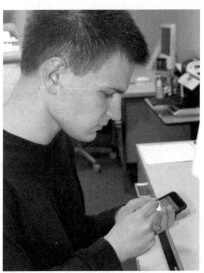

(Fig. 11-4) After completing a word processing task, Chris checks his schedule on his pocket computer.

was initially taught to take a break at an unoccupied table. His written schedule included the following tasks: get a magazine; get a diet soda; go to the lunch room; say "Hi" or "Hello" to people; sit down at a table; set wristwatch timer for ten minutes; look at magazine; when timer rings, go back to work. George's job coach covertly observed him and later gave him a snack of his choice if he did not engage in any stereotypic or inappropriate behavior during break. But if problem behavior was observed, the job coach quickly entered the lunch room, went to George's table, and quietly said, "Break is over—let's go back to work." George soon mastered his break schedule and looked very competent in the lunch room.

Ari and Jane work in the same corporation and eat lunch together in the employee cafeteria. Previously, each brought a written list of topics to the table; these lists, developed by their job coach, guided their lunchtime conversation. Now, their job coach enters lists of topics on the notes applications on their cell phones to cue social interaction. When Jane and Ari occasionally glance at their cell phones, they look like many other young adults in the cafeteria.

Problem Solving at Work

Although they may be skilled at completing their usual employment responsibilities, adults with autism may arrive at an impasse when unforeseen problems arise. Problem-solving schedules provide options when workers with autism encounter the unexpected.

Charles is employed as a file clerk in an investment company. He obtains files for his supervisors and returns files to designated locations. He was hired only a few months ago, and although he makes virtually no filing errors, he sometimes encounters problems that he cannot solve—for example, if a file he was asked to obtain is absent, or if a document to be filed does not match any name in the file cabinets.

These problems can often be resolved with activity schedules. Charles's work notebook is divided into sections and each section contains a written schedule. There is a schedule for taking breaks, a schedule for lunch in the cafeteria, and several sections about problem solving. For example, one section of the notebook is labeled "Can't find a file." The entries in this section include: Look for the file again; Ask your supervisor, "Is someone using the ____ file?"; Did the supervisor say, "Yes" or "No"? (Circle *yes* or *no*); If you circled *yes*, continue to file; if you circled *no*, call your job coach.

Problem-solving schedules teach useful work skills while helping many young workers achieve greater independence. Victor's work supervisor spoke English as a second language, and Victor was sometimes unable to understand him when he was given work assignments. A written schedule helped him learn to politely ask for clarification; then, if he still did not understand, his schedule directed him to call his job coach, and ask him to speak to

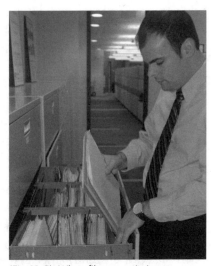

(Fig 11-5) When files are missing, Charles uses a problem-solving schedule.

the supervisor. After obtaining the relevant information, the job coach thanked the supervisor and gave Victor his work assignments.

Sometimes, even the most skilled workers with autism exhibit behavior problems that endanger their continued employment, but problem-solving schedules can prevent job loss. For example, Angela had a long history of tantrums, which had decreased in frequency with effective intervention. When she was employed in a data-entry position, however, she sometimes cried or spoke too loudly when she was disappointed (for example, her coffee break was delayed, her supervisor gave abrupt corrective feedback, or she forgot her lunch). Angela's job coach helped her learn to follow a problem-solving schedule that allowed her to express her disappointment in private. Her schedule directed her to leave her desk, go to the women's room, sit in a stall, set a timer, and reset the timer if necessary until she was calm, and then return to her desk. The schedule preserved her job, and her exceptional data-entry skills have been recognized in the company newsletter.

Activity schedules enable adults with autism to retain employment and succeed in community workplaces. Although workers with more severe developmental disabilities may need daily supervision, others pursue complex tasks in blue-collar and white-collar settings with every-other-day or twice-weekly visits from job coaches.

Activity Schedules in the Community

Activity schedules can be invaluable in promoting community integration for adolescents and adults with autism (Rehfeldt, 2002). For example, written or photographic schedules have helped many adults learn to use cell phones, giving them an additional measure of safety when they are in community settings. If a job coach has car trouble and must arrive late to provide transportation from work to home, he can call the worker with autism, explain the change of schedule, and suggest a good place for the worker to wait for his ride. If a young person becomes ill while at work, she can call someone to transport her from work to home. Cell phones are also helpful if a person who uses public transportation encounters a scheduling problem, takes the wrong train or bus and becomes lost, or is approached by a stranger. Learning to use a cell phone makes a key contribution to the safety of people with autism.

Many older children and teens use activity schedules to learn to make purchases (see Figure 11-6), and these schedules are later expanded to teach grocery and clothing shopping. Schedules are also helpful in teaching people to order in restaurants. Often, they first learn to place orders in fast-food establishments where there are fewer choices and tips are unnecessary; later, they learn to order in restaurants that offer expanded menus. A well-constructed schedule not only teaches people to place orders and request and pay the check, but also teaches them to be polite—to say "please" and "thank you," and to wait appropriately until food is served.

Using an automatic teller machine (ATM) is also taught via activity schedules. And because we want young workers to value their pay checks, we often help them plan special community outings (such as going to a movie, a sports event, or an amusement park) that occur soon after they deposit their checks and obtain cash from the ATM.

Activity schedules are also helpful in teaching people to use vending machines, calculate tips, balance checkbooks, pack a suitcase, and use laundromats (McClannahan, MacDuff, and Krantz, 2009).

Activity Schedules and Task Analyses

Making a task analysis means breaking a skill into specific responses or steps that are necessary to correctly perform the skill (Reid

Fig. 11-6 | A Written Activity Schedule for Making Purchases

_____ 1. Get billfold

_____ 2. Look in billfold for money

_____ 3. Tell someone, "I want to buy_____.

Do I have enough money?"

_____ 4. Put billfold in pocket or purse

_____ 5. Go in store and choose an item

_____ 6. Find cash register

_____ 7. Wait in line

_____ 8. Put item on counter

_____ 9. Get billfold

_____ 10. Give money to cashier

_____ 11. Wait for change

_____ 12. Take change

_____ 13. Put change in pocket, billfold, or purse

_____ 14. Say "Thank you"

_____ 15. Take item and leave store

and Green, 2005). Activity schedules are based on task analyses—the better the task analysis, the better the schedule.

Some task analyses are long (such as cleaning a hotel room), and others are quite short. For example, a task analysis of getting the mail may have only five steps:

1. go to the mailbox,
2. remove all of the mail from the box,
3. bring the mail to the house,
4. put the mail on the table in the hall, and
5. tell a family member, "I got the mail."

This task analysis could be used to create either a written or a photographic schedule. If we wanted to construct a photographic schedule, we might take a picture of the learner on his way to the mailbox, a picture of him removing the mail from the box, a picture of him returning to the house carrying the mail, a picture of him putting the mail on the hall table, and a picture of him interacting with a family member.

It's important to use task analyses to individualize the resulting activity schedules. One person may not need the written cue "bring the mail to the house," or a picture of himself returning to the house. But without that cue, another person may be unable to continue following the schedule. It may be important to one adult to add steps to a brownie recipe (get white measuring cup, get milk, pour milk into white cup, put milk in bowl), but another person may have learned to respond to more conventional parts of a recipe (add 1 cup milk).

Some components of task analyses are difficult to show in photographs. We may do a task analysis of tooth brushing because we want to create an activity schedule that helps a person do a better job of brushing his molars, but it is virtually impossible to take a photograph that shows the desired response. Further, people who use photographic schedules often do not understand concepts such as right and left, or upper and lower. Fortunately, in most cases, manual guidance and prompt-fading procedures teach people to respond to photographs or words that did not previously cue relevant behavior.

Task analyses can prevent or encourage errors in schedule following. Omission of any of several key components in Kate's e-mail schedule (see Figure 11-3) could make it impossible for her to carry on correspondence with friends and family members. Adding unnecessary components to an activity schedule may teach people *not* to follow the schedule if they skip steps because they have already learned them. But omitting responses that have not yet been acquired typically results in errors.

For these reasons, it is helpful if parents, instructors, and job coaches do task analyses by actually doing and recording the component tasks in the target skill. For example, before she makes the activity schedule, Mother should make the meatloaf and write down all of the steps that she believes her son will need if he is to be successful. The job coach should clean the hotel room and bathroom, record the required steps, and subsequently use the task analysis to individualize an activity schedule for each housekeeper with autism. Father should do a task analysis of playing billiards or using a putting green before making those schedules. And instructors should do and record target tasks and individualize activity schedules before teaching people to use exercise equipment; clip nails; take pills; or attend mosque, temple, or church.

When we use task analyses and individualize activity schedules, we expect that after some teaching, many adults will be able to complete several component responses without referring to their schedules. This is a signal that they are mastering the tasks—but we don't want them to learn that they don't need to use their schedules. Instead, we revise the schedules and delete the photographs or textual cues that are no longer needed. If we are good observers, and if we delete pictures or words that are no longer necessary, many activity schedules will eventually be reduced to a word or a few words that appear in a main schedule—such as "get ready for work," "make dinner," or "e-mail."

12 | Activity Schedules: A Platform for Progress

Schedules are not effective if they are used only for isolated activities, only in a few settings, or only for limited periods of time. If used regularly, across each day, they offer a framework that helps people with autism organize all aspects of their lives. Across the life span, schedules teach key repertoires, such as sustained engagement, task completion, making appropriate choices, sequencing activities, and pursuing many tasks without immediate supervision. Activity schedules should not be static, but fluid—they must change in form and specificity and grow with the learner.

Activity Schedules Increase Engagement

In the intervention programs we have helped to develop in the United States and other countries, every enrolled child or adult with autism uses an activity schedule, and their appropriate engagement with scheduled activities is very high. In all seven intervention programs, the data show that, on average, the young people with autism are on-task or engaged with planned activities on 80% to 100% of observations. These levels of engagement are higher than those often found in public school classrooms and day care centers for typical children. Many studies demonstrate that activity schedules increase on-task behavior (see Anderson, Sherman, Sheldon, & McAdam, 1997; Bryan & Gast, 2000; Krantz, MacDuff, & McClannahan, 1993; MacDuff, Krantz, & McClannahan, 1993; and Watanabe & Sturmey, 2003).

Activity Schedules Decrease Problem Behavior

All of us like to know the day's agenda. We want to know what meetings or appointments are scheduled, whether there are deadlines to be met, and which family members will be home for dinner. The same is true for many youngsters with autism. Disruptive behavior often decreases when a child's activity schedule reveals the events of the day and makes life more predictable. For example, Miles's parents reported that he often had tantrums preceding outdoor activities, but the tantrums ceased when his photographic activity schedule depicted the nature of the activity, such as bike riding or taking a car ride (Krantz, MacDuff, & McClannahan, 1993).

Sometimes disruptive behavior occurs because children have not yet acquired the skills needed to fill unstructured periods of time. Research showed that the challenging behavior of three school-age children with autism decreased during recess after they learned to follow a schedule of play activities (Machalicek, Shogren, Lang, Rispoli, O'Reilly, Franco, & Sigafoos, 2009).

Children (with and without autism) do not spend their waking hours "doing nothing." They are busy. They use the skills we have taught, respond to instructions, and develop additional skills, and in situations that are unclear, they often display unwanted behavior. Typical preschoolers who have not yet learned to manage unstructured time may hit a sibling, make repeated bids for attention when a parent is visiting with a friend, or have a tantrum when told that TV time is over. In the absence of structure, children with autism also have difficulty, but their unwanted responses may include stereotypy and self-injury. Learning to use activity schedules organizes their time and helps them know the agenda. In addition, the teaching procedures (especially manual guidance) prevent or abbreviate problem behavior that might otherwise be increasingly practiced and elaborated.

Activity Schedules Help Young People Learn to Learn

Children with autism must learn to learn in many different ways: from discrete-trial instruction; from incidental teaching; from television; from computer; from videotaped models; from parents, teachers, and peers; and from pictorial, auditory, and textual cues (Krantz, 2000). Activity schedules provide a framework that helps parents and teachers plan and include many different science-based procedures that help youngsters develop new skills. For example, discrete-trial instruction may be included in a preschooler's schedule to help him learn to imitate words. His activity schedule displays a photograph of him and his teacher sitting face-to-face at a little table; a button-activated recorder that is attached to the photo plays the script, "talk." The child removes the picture and voice recorder from his schedule, approaches and orients toward the teacher, presses the button to play the message, and then approximates the word "talk." His teacher responds, "It's fun to talk to you!" and gives him a token. Then she conducts a verbal imitation session.

Similarly, an instructor may include incidental teaching in a girl's schedule to help her learn to request assistance. As a first lesson, the girl's favorite snacks (gummy bears and Ritz Bits) are placed in transparent containers with screw-on lids. The containers are photographed and the pictures are interspersed in the activity schedule. When the girl turns to a page that shows one of these photos, she gets the container from the shelf, but is unable to open it. The teacher approaches and suggests, "Say, 'Please help me.'" The girl responds, the teacher confirms that the student's response was correct ("Good, you said, 'Please help me'") and removes the lid and provides access to the preferred snack.

In another example, a young girl with minimal play skills turns a page and points to a picture of doll clothing and a toy iron and ironing board. She removes a voice recorder from the page, approaches her teacher, presses the button, and says the now-faded script, "Time to iron." The teacher says, "You can iron the doll's dresses," and they move to a play area that contains a TV and DVD player and a toy iron and ironing board. The teacher plays a video scenario showing play with the toys, and the girl imitates the motor and verbal models; she pretends to iron, and imitates scripts such as "The iron is hot" and "This dress is pretty."

There are many well-researched intervention procedures that address diverse instructional objectives. Activity schedules can include all of them.

Activity Schedules Foster Independence

Young people who are skilled schedule users don't wait for adults to tell them what to do; they identify next activities and when appropriate, approach parents, teachers, peers, or siblings with initiations such as, "It's time for spelling," "Could you check my work?" or "Want to shoot baskets?" They obtain necessary materials, complete activities, and put things away without being told. And if prompt-fading procedures are correctly and systematically used, they complete previously mastered tasks without ongoing supervision. Below are several examples of ways that activity schedules lead to increased independence for young people with autism.

An eight-year-old turns a page of his schedule and finds a picture of a classroom computer. He goes to the computer, opens the Type to Learn program, opens his own data file, practices keyboard skills, completes a lesson, saves his work, and returns to his schedule. Manual guidance and prompt fading enabled him to do this chain of responses without help.

A twelve-year-old places a checkmark beside a completed activity in her written schedule; the next item on her schedule is the card game Uno. She obtains the cards, goes to the family room where her younger brother is watching television, and says, "Let's play Uno." Her mother, who has been covertly observing from the kitchen, calls, "Would you two like some popcorn while you play cards?"

A teenager's after-school schedule includes the text, "Empty wastebaskets." As he pursues this activity, he accidentally knocks over a basket, spilling the contents. He carefully picks up all of the items that fell on the floor and then continues the task.

Activity Schedules Promote Skill Generalization

There is a body of evidence showing that when activity schedules are taught with manual guidance and a most-to-least prompt-fading sequence, pictures and textual cues come to evoke generalized responding. That is, schedule following skills transfer to different sequences of pictures and to new pictures; they generalize across persons; they generalize across settings—for example, from school or group home to home—and they generalize across tasks.

During a six-month period, we assessed the skill generalization of eight students with autism, ages 12 to 17. Their scores on standardized tests ranged from severely to moderately disabled and all of them were experienced schedule followers. For each new teaching program introduced during the study period, two pretests were administered—the first without and the second with an activity schedule. During the pretests, the instructor gave one initial direction (for example, "Please make potato-tuna salad" or "Please clean the mirror and sink"), after which no prompts were delivered. On 30 of 32 new programs (94%) introduced, the students achieved higher pretest scores when activity schedules were present than when they were absent. The magnitude of difference ranged from 3% to 75% more tasks correctly completed. This study demonstrated that schedule-following skills generalized to new, never-taught schedules that targeted a variety of activities, such as food preparation, housekeeping tasks, and personal hygiene activities, and skill generalization was observed for students with severe as well as moderate disabilities (McClannahan, MacDuff, & Krantz, 2009). Skill generalization promotes rapid acquisition, opening new avenues to next achievements.

Activity Schedules Help Young People Use the Same Cues We Use

For more than twenty years we have helped people with autism (toddlers, school-age children, and adults) learn to use activity schedules, and we have never yet met a person who could not acquire these skills. Skill acquisition takes longer for some than for others; some learners do not develop reading skills and continue to use photographic schedules in adulthood. Others ultimately use agendas that are identical to yours and mine. All benefit from learning to follow schedules.

People make minimal progress if schedules remain the same for long periods of time. They make more progress if we persist in adjusting and re-designing their schedules as they develop new skills. As soon as possible, the four or five photographs in a toddler's schedule should be re-sequenced, and then additional photographs should be added. The number of activities in the schedule should be expanded, and choices should be introduced. Tangible rewards given during schedule following should gradually be replaced by token rewards that are exchanged at the end of the schedule.

Young readers should move on to written to-do lists, even though some of the words must be separately taught in discrete-trial sessions before they are added to schedules. Next, to-do lists should appear in planners or DayTimers and then youngsters should begin to sequence their own activities. Schedules should be systematically extended, so that they are used for more and more hours at school, at home, and in the community. Mastered tasks, previously represented by many pictures or words, should be replaced by a single photograph or a few words (for example, a picture of a breakfast, or the words "clean my room"). For many people, planners should be supplanted by pocket computers that present either photographic or textual cues. Take a quick look around; in many contemporary environments, many people are using PDAs and cell phones. Young people with autism who use hand-held computers look just like the rest of us. (Or they may look like others of us—probably a shrinking minority—who continue to prefer handwritten to-do lists or planners.)

In a better world, people with disabilities would always receive respect and equal treatment. Unfortunately, in today's world, they sometimes encounter prejudice, discrimination, and social disapproval. Learning to use organizational systems and cues similar to those used by everyone else can help others view them as competent employees and valued participants in community life.

13 | Problem Solving

Introduction

Many parents and teachers who help young people with autism learn to use activity schedules report some difficulties along the way. Teaching can be demanding, and it isn't always smooth sailing. This chapter discusses some frequently posed questions and concerns, and offers suggestions about how to deal with problems that are sometimes encountered during teaching.

He seems bored with the schedule.

Neither we nor young people with autism like to work on difficult tasks. But after we become proficient, we enjoy using and displaying our skills. If we want children to enjoy playing with toys, coloring, doing arithmetic worksheets, making snacks, or initiating interactions with others, we must provide multiple practice opportunities. If your son appears uninterested in activities that he has not yet mastered, continue to use the manual guidance and prompt-fading procedures until he meets the accuracy criteria. Later, after he masters the skills, he may choose the activities that presently appear difficult or uninteresting.

Of course, when any learning problem is noted, it is always a good idea to review the available rewards, and to substitute new snacks, toys, games, or social activities for those that no longer appear interesting. If the child is exchanging his tokens for Cheerios, try a different snack. If his schedule includes a toss in the air, consider replacing that activity with a "swing your partner" or "hang upside down" game. And as noted in Chapter 6, don't wait too long to change the order of activities in the schedule, or to introduce new activities.

She makes vocal noise or engages in motor stereotypy while doing her schedule.

One of the reasons for teaching schedule following is to help your child acquire new skills that are incompatible with vocal or motor stereotypy. If she hums, coos, repeats the same sound, or says a word or phrase over and over, remember that typical children are seldom silent during work and play activities. Continue to teach, but be especially careful not to provide snacks, tokens, or other special rewards when she is displaying repetitive behavior.

If she attempts to engage in hand flapping, finger play, hand regarding, rocking, or other stereotyped motor behavior, return to manual guidance to prevent this behavior. The occurrence of repetitive motor responses is often predictable—one child may display stereotypic head turning each time she picks up laminated picture cards, another may flap her hands whenever a musical toy is activated, and a third may exhibit finger play before or after turning a page in the schedule book. If you can predict the onset of stereotypy, you can use manual guidance to prevent it. If it reappears after you move to spatial fading, take this as an indication that fading began too soon and return to graduated guidance. Even if you can't predict and prevent dysfunctional motor responses, you can interrupt them quickly, so that there is little time to practice them.

He sometimes tantrums when we are teaching him to use his schedule.

It is unlikely that your son will learn much about his schedule while he is having a tantrum, and you probably don't want to risk having tantrum behavior become part of the new response sequences he is learning, so it's best to stop the schedule and do whatever you usually do about tantrums. (For example, put him in a high chair, in his room, or on the bottom stair step until he is quiet and ready to follow directions.)

If tantrums occur frequently, reevaluate the rewards embedded in the schedule, and consider increasing the frequency of delivery of tokens, snacks, or especially enjoyable activities when he is performing well. But be careful not to teach him that having a tantrum prevents him from having to do his schedule. When the tantrum is over, began the schedule again.

Activity schedules are most effective when used throughout children's waking hours. If a youngster is asked to follow a five-page activity schedule, but during the remainder of the day his parents make few requests and allow him to engage in stereotypic and ritualistic behavior, it is likely that he will display disruptive behavior when asked to follow the schedule. Similarly, if a youngster has two hours of discrete-trial instruction per day, during which he is rewarded for every correct response, he may resist making several schedule-following responses (such as obtaining and completing a puzzle and putting it away) before receiving a reward. It is important to make schedule following as rewarding as other daily activities.

She takes pennies before she earns them.

Children must learn that they may not take things that do not rightfully belong to them. Using token rewards is one way to teach your child this important principle, which will help her earn others' respect. Use manual guidance to prevent your youngster from taking coins, snacks, or other rewards not yet earned. But if she responds so quickly that you can't prevent her from grabbing a token, immediately remove it. If this behavior continues, you may decide not only to recover the token she grabbed, but to remove several additional coins or stickers and avoid giving her the number of tokens she needs in order to purchase the final snack or special activity.

Not uncommonly, children cooperate with token delivery during graduated guidance or spatial fading, but start to "steal" tokens when parents begin shadowing or decreasing their physical proximity. This is a signal to return, at least temporarily, to the prior prompting procedure. When you once again begin to fade prompts, your child's behavior will tell you whether to continue the fading procedures.

My son has learned to use his schedule, but I have to stay in the room with him.

As noted in Chapter 6 (see New Problems, Familiar Solutions), fading adult proximity is perhaps the most difficult step in helping a child achieve real independence. Many children learn to follow several different schedules before they learn to pursue previously mastered activities in the absence of parents or teachers.

If, after learning several schedules, your child is not successful when you are outside the room, there are several strategies you may explore. Try decreasing your proximity while engaging in another activity such as reading, folding laundry, or interacting with another family member. Although you continue to covertly observe his performance so that you can step in to prompt if needed, your scrutiny may be less relevant to him.

In addition, if your child is verbal, you may want to include more social interaction tasks in his schedule, especially interactions that focus on task completion. Teach him to report to you after he completes each scheduled activity—for example, "I did puzzle" or "I made cheese crackers"—and praise and reward him for his independent work (or withhold praise and rewards if he completed the activity with prompts). Gradually move farther away when it is time for him to report, so that he must eventually come to find you in another room.

Finally, move out of his sight for only a few seconds at a time, and time your return so that you can reward him for remaining engaged when you are absent. Then very gradually increase the number of seconds when you are not visible to him.

Of course, some scheduled activities are designed to be done in the presence of parents. Some youngsters' schedules include cues such as "Ask Dad to check my homework," or "Tell Mom it's time for language," or "Ask for help with arithmetic." Such scheduled activities create a platform for additional teaching—a parent may offer feedback on handwriting worksheets, provide discrete-trail training on articulation, or present flash cards that help the child memorize addition facts.

If you use your son's schedule to remind you to review his homework assignments or help him with speech, you can maintain his growing independence by making him responsible for obtaining and putting away materials. Instead of telling him that it's time to put things away, simply indicate that the activity is over (e.g., "You're done with homework" or "We're finished with flash cards").

I can't always be home to do her schedule with her. Can I change it?

Some of us accept schedule changes better than others, but all of us must show some flexibility. Changes in work schedules, changes in family members' commitments, and unexpected events often require us to juggle responsibilities and revise our plans. By teaching your daughter to use an activity schedule, you can teach her to tolerate changes in routine.

When necessary, don't hesitate to abbreviate your child's photographic or written schedule. If you must run errands or take another child to an after-school event, remove several pages from her schedule book and substitute a page that indicates a car ride. And after you have resequenced activities and she has mastered more than one schedule, feel free to add new components when this will help you respond to other obligations.

If you can anticipate certain schedule changes, prepare pictorial or textual cues in advance and provide practice opportunities when the daily routine is relatively forgiving. For example, add photographs that indicate meeting a parent at the train or bus station; taking a sibling to soccer practice; going to the mall, to the pediatrician, or to grandma's house; watching TV; bathing; or going to bed. From time to time, delete some usual activities and add these alternate activities, even when circumstances do not require that you do so. This will not only contribute to the quality of life of other family members, but will also help your youngster with autism learn to accept change and make positive contributions to your family.

An activity schedule is merely a tool. Make ongoing decisions about your daughter's daily schedule, just as you make decisions about other aspects of her education and family participation.

We're so busy that I can hardly find time to set up his schedule each day.

As a parent of a child with autism, you have learned many coping skills that help you deal with the demands of everyday life. Teaching your son to use an activity schedule initially increases those demands, but ultimately creates some freedom for you. Some advance attention to the design of his work and play environment will help you reap these rewards. Chapter 3 discusses arrangements of materials that contribute to young people's independence.

Given a well-designed learning environment, you can not only teach your child to use an activity schedule, but also to take responsibility for his possessions. If there is a designated place for work and play materials, the teaching procedures will enable him to put things away. When you begin a new schedule, don't hesitate to manually guide him to do a few "extra" activities that are not shown in the photographs or elaborated in the text. If he builds a K'Nex model, guide him to disassemble it and put the pieces back in the bin before he puts it away. If he cuts with scissors, guide him to pick up scraps of paper and throw them in the wastebasket. If he makes pudding, teach him to finish by wiping the counter and putting utensils in the dishwasher.

Ultimately, activity schedules are only useful if we use the teaching procedures to enable children to exhibit criterion performances; that is, to complete target activities skillfully and correctly, so that others don't have to accept inadequate performances or re-do tasks later. Learning to make meatloaf is a functional skill only if the activity does not create more work for others, and if the meatloaf tastes good and contributes to the family dinner. Learning to vacuum the carpet is useful only if the carpet is clean at the end of the activity. And learning to use an activity schedule is most useful when young people learn to manage their own schedules and materials. All of these important outcomes are accomplished by using the teaching procedures described earlier.

I'm worried that the activity schedule is adding to my child's social isolation.

Some young schedule users appear very engrossed in planned activities, and may even ignore others who are nearby. Many children, like us, prefer not to be interrupted during nonsocial tasks such as using the computer, reading or looking at books or magazines, completing worksheets, or cooking. But if your child attempts to isolate herself during social activities—for example, avoids looking at you while talking to you, or while receiving a tickle—you may want to add more social activities to her schedule and provide rewards only when she interacts and looks at others. As noted earlier, social interaction is a key deficit for children with autism. Multiple practice opportunities, followed by powerful rewards, help build social competence.

In fact, well-designed activity schedules decrease social isolation. Activity schedules shouldn't involve special "therapy rooms"—the whole house and yard, the school, the car, and the community are instructional settings. If your child hasn't yet learned to use a schedule without adult supervision, teach her to use a play schedule while sitting on a small rug that defines the boundaries of the activity area. Move the rug and schedule to the living room when family members are watching television, to the laundry room while you fold clothes, and to her grandparents' house during visits there. Make activity schedules for her that are parallel to your daily activities. Teach her to use a schedule for setting the table and preparing her school lunch while you prepare dinner. Prepare a schedule that she can follow when her siblings are doing homework, and add some activities that cue her to interact with them.

My child seems to want manual guidance all of the time. How can I fade prompts?

Many youngsters with autism appear to enjoy physical contact, perhaps because of parents' efforts to draw them into a social world. And some children wait to be manually guided because they have learned to depend upon adults' prompts (see Chapter 4—Why Manual Guidance?). If your child waits to be prompted, magnify your physical contact with him. Consider adding tickling, wrestling, hugging, and roughhousing, both as scheduled activities, and as rewards that are earned at the end of the schedule. Deliver a minimum of these activities when he waits to be prompted, and offer intensive, lengthy physical contact when he is performing well.

Our preschooler has trouble turning the pages of her schedule.

It's not unusual for a child to develop schedule-following skills before acquiring the manual dexterity needed to turn pages, and it's quite acceptable to devise temporary alternatives. Some youngsters learn to use large tabs attached to the right side of each page, enabling them to turn one page at a time. Others succeed at page turning if we attach Velcro to the bottom of each page. (This separates pages, making it easier to grasp a single page.)

My son still doesn't have picture-object correspondence skills. What should I do?

Learning picture-object correspondence is sometimes a major hurdle. We have known children who mastered this skill only after several years of instruction. In the meantime, we bypassed the issue and helped them become schedule users by focusing on their matching skills. If a youngster can match pictures, put one picture in his schedule book and attach an identical picture to a bin that contains the relevant materials. If he can match alphabet letters or numerals, put letters or numerals in his schedule book and attach corresponding letters or numerals to baskets that contain toys or learning activities. If he hasn't yet learned to match two-dimensional pictures but can match objects, mount objects in his book and on containers. For example, put a real puzzle piece in his book, and attach an identical puzzle piece to the puzzle container. We know youngsters who learned to take bathroom breaks or ride tricycles when doll-furniture toilets and trikes were attached to schedule pages. Continue to work on picture-object correspondence—these skills make important contributions to independence.

How long should we wait before we prompt?

We often feel impaled on the horns of this dilemma. If we prompt too soon, we prevent a young person from enjoying independent task completion. If we prompt too late, she may make an error that will appear again and again. When to prompt is a judgment that each of us must make on the basis of our previous observations. If she usually completes this task independently, it is likely that she will do that again, even after a pause of ten or fifteen seconds. If this is a difficult task (one that usually requires assistance), prompt quickly, before she forgets what she is doing or engages in an inappropriate behavior. Observation of her current performance offers the best guidelines about when to prompt.

Ken

We have known Ken since he was three, and autism is only one of his diagnoses. He has severe developmental disabilities, takes seizure-control medications that often produce undesirable side effects, and has long-standing health problems. Now forty years old, he did not learn to follow a photographic activity schedule until he was sixteen, when this technology became available, but it made an important difference in his life. His daily schedule cues him to do personal hygiene tasks, to help with household chores such as setting the table and cleaning his room, and to choose leisure activities. At work, his schedule helps him count and package parts used in the automotive industry, and enables him to select among a variety of options about how to spend break time. Social interactions are included in Ken's schedule, and although his vocabulary is limited, he enthusiastically approaches others to discuss his plans for days off, for visiting relatives, or going to favorite restaurants. He is pleasant and productive, and we look forward to our conversations with him. Although we can't measure happiness, he appears to us to be happy.

Appendices

Appendix A   Prerequisite Sills Data Sheets

Prerequisite Skills Data Sheet for _____

Opportunity#	Task	Date/Time	Date/Time	Date/Time
	Picture Versus Background			
1				
2				
3				
4				
5				
6				
7				
8				
9				
10				
Number Correct				

Opportunity#	Task	Date/Time	Date/Time	Date/Time
	Matching Identical Objects			
1				
2				
3				
4				
5				
6				
7				
8				
9				
10				
Number Correct				

Opportunity#	Task	Date/Time	Date/Time	Date/Time
	Picture-Object Correspondence			
1				
2				
3				
4				
5				
Number Correct				

Appendix B   Button-Activated Voice Recorders

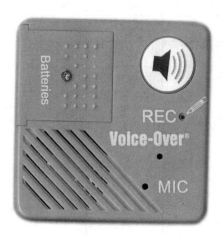
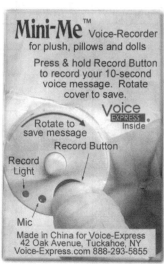

These miniature voice recorders may be ordered from:
 ARGUS Media LLC
 90 Shetland Road
 Fairfield, CT 06824
 203-254-3503; 203-254-3581 (fax)
 or
 Alexander's Shoppe
 www.teachwithsound.com

At the time of publication, Mini-Mes were $6.20 each, and Voice-Overs were $6.50 each.

Appendix C Audio Card Readers

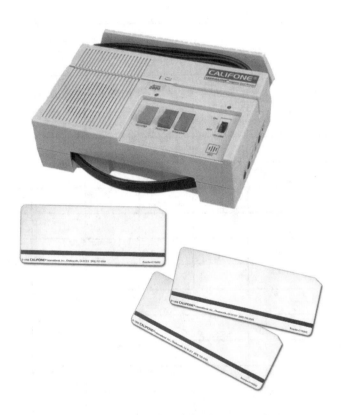

` Califone card readers may be ordered from:
    Cousins Video
    420 W. Prospect Street
    Painesville, OH 44077
    800-256-5977; 440-354-0651 (fax)
    info@cousinsvideo.com
    www.cousinsvideo.com

At the time of publication, card reader model 2010AV listed for $173.80, and 100 blank cards were $32.60.

Appendix D   Schedule Following Data Sheets

OBSERVER:					
DATE:					
Activity	Opens Book/ Turns Page	Points/ Looks	Obtains	Completes	Puts Away
# Completed					
Number of components correctly completed:					
Total number of components:					
Percentage of components correctly completed:					

OBSERVER:

DATE:

Activity	Opens Book/ Turns Page	Points/ Looks	Obtains	Completes	Puts Away
# Completed					

Number of components correctly completed:

Total number of components:

Percentage of components correctly completed:

References

Anderson, M. D., Sherman, J. A., Sheldon, J. B., & McAdam, D. (1997). Picture activity schedules and engagement of adults with mental retardation in a group home. *Research in Developmental Disabilities, 18*, 231-50.

Betz, A., Higbee, T. S., & Reagon, K. A. (2008). Using joint activity schedules to promote peer engagement in preschoolers with autism. *Journal of Applied Behavior Analysis, 41*, 237-41.

Birkan, B., McClannahan, L. E., & Krantz, P. J. (2007). Effects of superimposition and background fading on the sight-word reading of a boy with autism. *Research in Autism Spectrum Disorders, 1*, 117-25.

Bryan, L. C. & Gast, D. L. (2000). Teaching on-task and on-schedule behaviors to high-functioning children with autism via picture activity schedules. *Journal of Autism and Developmental Disorders, 30*, 553-67.

Cooper, J. O. (1987). Stimulus control. In J. O. Cooper, T. E. Heron, & W. L. Heward, *Applied Behavior Analysis* (p. 315). Columbus, OH: Merrill Publishing Co.

Decker, D.M., Ferrigno, T. K., May D. T., Natoli, C. L., Olson, K. D., Schaefer, M. A., Cammilleri, A. P., & Brothers, K. J. (2003, May). *A comparison of student performance on paper and electronic picture activity schedules.* Poster presented at the First Annual Conference of the Princeton Child Development Institute, Princeton, NJ.

Edmark Corporation (1992). *Edmark Reading Program.* Redmond, WA: Author.

Etzel, B. C. & LeBlanc, J. M. (1979). The simplest treatment alternative: The law of parsimony applied to choosing appropriate instructional control and errorless-learning procedures for the difficult-to-teach child. *Journal of Autism and Developmental Disorders, 9,* 361-382.

Krantz, P. J. (2000). Commentary: Interventions to facilitate socialization. *Journal of Autism and Developmental Disorders, 30,* 411-413.

Krantz, P. J., MacDuff, M. T., & McClannahan, L. E. (1993). Programming participation in family activities for children with autism: Parents' use of photographic activity schedules. *Journal of Applied Behavior Analysis, 26,* 137-139.

Krantz, P. J. & McClannahan, L. E. (1993). Teaching children with autism to initiate to peers: Effects of a script-fading procedure. *Journal of Applied Behavior Analysis, 26,* 121-132.

Krantz, P. J. & McClannahan, L. E. (1998). Social interaction skills for children with autism: A script-fading procedure for beginning readers. *Journal of Applied Behavior Analysis, 31,* 191-202.

Lovaas, O. I. (1977). *The autistic child: Language development through behavior modification.* New York: Irvington.

Lutzker, J. R., McGimsey-McRae, S., & McGimsey, J. F. (1983). General description of behavioral approaches. In M. Hersen, V. B. VanHasselt, & J. L. Matson (Eds.), *Behavior therapy for the developmentally and physically disabled* (p. 42). New York, NY: Academic Press.

MacDuff, G. S., Krantz, P. J., & McClannahan, L. E. (1993). Teaching children with autism to use photographic activity schedules: Maintenance and generalization of complex response chains. *Journal of Applied Behavior Analysis, 26,* 89-97.

Machalicek, W., Shogren, K., Lang, R., Rispoli, M., O'Reilly, M. F., Franco, J. H., & Sigafoos, J. (2009). Increasing play and decreasing the challenging behavior of children with autism during recess with activity schedules and task correspondence training. *Research in Autism Spectrum Disorders, 3,* 547-555.

McClannahan, L. E. (1998). From photographic to textual cues. In P. J. Krantz, G. S. MacDuff, E. C. Fenske, & L. E. McClannahan, *Teaching independence and choice: Design, implementation, and assessment of the use of activity schedules*. Princeton, NJ: Princeton Child Development Institute. DVDs or VHS tapes. www.pcdi.org

McClannahan, L. E. & Krantz, P. J. (1997). In search of solutions to prompt dependence: Teaching children with autism to use photographic activity schedules. In E. M. Pinkston and D. M. Baer (Eds.), *Environment and Behavior* (pp. 271-278). Boulder, CO: Westview Press.

McClannahan, L. E. & Krantz, P. J. (2005). *Teaching conversation to children with autism: Scripts and script fading*. Bethesda, MD: Woodbine House.

McClannahan, L. E., MacDuff, G. S., & Krantz, P. J. (2002). Behavior analysis and intervention for adults with autism. *Behavior Modification, 26*, 9-26.

McClannahan, L. E., MacDuff, G. S., & Krantz, P. J. (2009). Activity schedules for adults with autism spectrum disorders. In P. Reed (Ed.), *Behavioral Theories and Interventions for Autism* (pp. 313-334). New York, NY: Nova Science Publishers.

McGee, G. G., Krantz, P. J., & McClannahan, L. E. (1986). An extension of incidental teaching procedures to reading instruction for autistic children. *Journal of Applied Behavior Analysis, 19*, 147-157.

Mechling, L. C., Gast, D. L., & Seid, N. H. (2009).Using a personal digital assistant to increase independent task completion by students with autism spectrum disorder. *Journal of Autism and Developmental Disorders, 39*, 1420-1434.

Miguel, C. F., Yang, H. G., Finn, H. E., & Ahearn, W. H. (2009). Establishing derived textual control in activity schedules with children with autism. *Journal of Applied Behavior Analysis, 42*, 703-709.

Pierce, K. L. & Schreibman, L. (1994). Teaching daily living skills to children with autism in unsupervised settings through pictorial self-management. *Journal of Applied Behavior Analysis, 27*, 471-481.

Rehfeldt, R. A. (2002). A review of McClannahan and Krantz's Activity schedules for children with autism: teaching independent behavior: Toward the inclusion and integration of children with disabilities. *The Behavior Analyst, 25*, 103-108.

Rehfeldt, R. A., Kinney, E. M., Root, S., & Stromer, R. (2004). Creating activity schedules using Microsoft PowerPoint. *Journal of Applied Behavior Analysis, 37*, 115-28.

Reid, D.H. & Green, C.W. (2005). *Preference-based Teaching: Helping People with Developmental Disabilities Enjoy Learning without Problem Behavior.* Morganton, NC: Habilitative Management Consultants.

Silver Lining Multimedia, Inc. (2008). *Picture This...* Poughkeepsie, NY: Author. (CD for Windows or Mac OS). www.silverliningmm.com

Stages Learning Materials (2009). *Language Builder: Picture Noun Cards.* Chico, CA: Author. www.stageslearning.com

Stevenson, C. L., Krantz, P. J., & McClannahan, L. E. (1998). Social interaction skills for children with autism: A script-fading procedure for nonreaders. *Behavioral Interventions, 15*, 1-20.

Watanabe, M. & Sturmey, P. (2003). The effect of choice-making opportunities during activity schedules on task engagement of adults with autism. *Journal of Autism and Developmental Disorders, 33*, 535-538.

Wichnick, A., Vener, S. M., Keating, C., & Poulson, C. L. (2010). The effect of a script-fading procedure on unscripted social initiations and novel utterances among young children with autism. *Research in Autism Spectrum Disorders, 4*, 51-64.

Index

Page numbers in italics indicate figures.

About the Authors

Lynn E. McClannahan, Ph.D. is Executive Director Emerita of the Princeton Child Development Institute, one of the first non-institutional programs in the United States for people with autism. Dr. McClannahan's work has been widely recognized by organizations such as the Senate of the State of New Jersey; the American Psychological Association; and the New Jersey Association for Behavior Analysis. With Dr. Krantz, she developed an intervention model that is used in the United States and abroad.

Patricia J. Krantz, Ph.D. is Executive Director Emerita of the Princeton Child Development Institute. Her research focuses on procedures that increase independence, choice, and spontaneous generative language. She is the author of many research articles and book chapters, and has made international contributions to autism intervention in Australia, Belgium, France, Norway, Poland, Russia, Spain, and Turkey, as well as in the United States. She and Dr. McClannahan continue to develop new intervention options for young people with autism.